This Book Can Mean The Very Breath of Life to You!

New Edition! Enlarged and Revise

BRAGG
SUPER POWER
BREATHING
for Super Health & High Energy

PAUL C. BRAGG, N.D., Ph.D.
LIFE EXTENSION SPECIALIST
and
PATRICIA BRAGG, N.D., Ph.D.
LIFE EXTENSION NUTRITIONIST

Health   Peace
Happiness   Youthfulness
Love   Joy
Praise   Patience
Vitality   Fortitude
Strength   Charity
Faith

JOIN

The Bragg Crusades for a 100% Healthy, Better World for All!

HEALTH SCIENCE
Box 7, Santa Barbara, CA 93102 USA
World Wide Web: http://www.bragg.com

BRAGG

SUPER POWER
BREATHING

for Super Health, High Energy & Longevity
Formerly: Super Brain Breathing

PAUL C. BRAGG, N.D., Ph.D.
and
PATRICIA BRAGG, N.D., Ph.D.

**To order Bragg Books and products on-line, visit our
World Wide Web site at: http://www.bragg.com**

Quantity Purchases: Companies, Professional Groups, Churches, Clubs, etc. please contact our Special Sales Department.

- New Edition – Enlarged and Revised -
Copyright © Health Science
Formerly: Bragg Super Brain Breathing

Sixteenth printing MCMXCV
ISBN: 0-87990-019-1

Published in the United States by
HEALTH SCIENCE - Box 7, Santa Barbara, Calif. 93102, USA

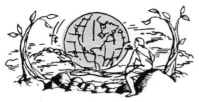

CHAPTER 2

CONTENTS

To preserve health is a moral and religious duty, for health is the basis for all social virtues. We can no longer be useful when not well.
                                        – Dr. Samuel Johnson, Father of Dictionaries

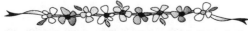

Of all the knowledge, that most worth having is knowledge about health. The first requisite of a good life is to be a healthy person. – Herbert Spencer

The best way to lengthen life is to avoid shortening it.

Fasting is the greatest remedy; the physician within. – Paracelsus
15th century physician who established the role of chemistry in medicine.

Paul Bragg's work on fasting is one of the great contributions to healing wisdom and the Natural Health Movement in the world today.
– Gabriel Cousens, M.D., Author *Conscious Eating and Spiritual Nutrition*

BRAGG CRUSADES For The 1990s
Teaching People World-Wide To Live
Healthier, Stronger Lives For A Better World

We love sharing, teaching and giving and you can share this love by being part of Bragg Crusades World-Wide Outreach. Bragg Crusades is dedicated to helping others. We feel blessed when your life improves from our teachings in the Bragg Books and Crusades. It makes our years of service so worthwhile!

The Miracle of Fasting book has been the No. 1 book for 10 years now in Russia. Why? Because we show them how to live a healthy, wholesome life for less money, and it's so easy to understand and follow. Most healthful lifestyle habits are free (examples - deep breathing, exercise, clean thoughts, good posture and plain, natural foods). We are continuing with all our health teachings, lectures, Crusades, radio, TV and video outreaches to reach the multitudes.

My joy and priorities come from God and healthy living. I'm excited about spreading health world-wide, for now it's needed more than ever. My father and I were also TV Health Pioneers, with our program "Health and Happiness" filmed in Hollywood. It's thrilling to be a Health Crusader and you will enjoy it also.

By reading the Bragg Self-Health Books you can also gain a new confidence that you are helping yourself, family & friends to Healthy Principles of Living! Please call your local health store & book store and ask for the Bragg Books. We hope to have all the stores stock the Bragg Books so they will be available to all.

I have visions of **Health Retreats** where people can find radiant health, joy and rebirth! They **will be Recharging - Physically, Mentally, Emotionally and Spiritually.** I was reared on Retreats ... holidays and vacations were spent at Camp for precious weeks of growth and recharge. You'll love them, too!

For the 1990s, we are planning Bragg Recharge Retreats, also Child & Senior Care Centers which are desperately needed across America. We are just waiting for the right locations and funding. We can accept all gifts, monetary and land (appraised value), and we can give a receipt for tax deductions. We could develop seldom-used ranches, farms and old estates into Recharge Centers for rejuvenating mind, body and soul. Those attending would become health crusaders for their families and friends. Empty buildings and spacious older homes with yards would make ideal Child & Senior Care Centers. Those who have any locations and who would like to be part of this great outreach, please write to me.

We are not new to retreats; my Dad pioneered the first health spa (Macfadden's Deauville) in Miami Beach and others in Highland Springs, CA and Danville, NY.

I expend all my energy and funds helping others to help themselves! Genuine love seeks ways to express itself! I thank you for your caring, sharing, support. For with your help we can achieve our goals for the 1990s. I know God will bless you. Your needed help will be a blessing to the Bragg Crusades. Our 1990s budget is for a mighty worthwhile cause. I know you, your family and friends will enjoy and benefit from the teachings and retreats.

With A Loving, Grateful Heart,   *Patricia Bragg*

BRAGG CRUSADES, America's Health Pioneers

A non-profit charitable organization. Gifts are tax deductible.
7340 Hollister Ave., Santa Barbara, CA 93117 USA (805) 968-1020
Over 80 continuous years spreading health and fitness worldwide.

Bragg
Super Power Breathing

Chapter 1

Do You Know How To Breathe?

The breath of life means exactly what it says. To breathe is to live. Not to breathe is to die. A human being can exist without food for weeks . . . without water for days . . . but without air he cannot exist for even a few minutes.

This fact is so obvious and breathing is so automatic that most people simply take it for granted. *But do you really know how to breathe?* Stop and think about it for a moment. Do you really know how your lungs function? Do you use these marvelous organs to their fullest capacity? The way you use your lungs controls your health. . . your looks . . . the way you feel . . . your resistance to disease . . . your very life span!

SUPER POWER BREATHING IS HIGH VIBRATION LIVING

As life extension specialists for well over half a century, we have developed techniques for measuring mental and physical energy in humans. Everyone lives at a certain rate of vibration. Unfortunately, very few live at the high vibration rate of which the human body is capable, because only a few know how to generate, utilize and replenish their full capacity of energy.

These high vibration people are the doers. They display seemingly inexhaustible vitality and stamina, creative power and/or athletic ability of the highest quality. They never seem to tire. They perform mental and physical tasks without strain, tension and excessive emotion. To high vibration achievers everything seems to be easy.

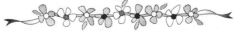

There is no substitute for Good Health.
Those who possess it are richer than kings.
– Paul C. Bragg

1

Above all, they are happy, contented people who always seem to find the humorous side of life. They are full of personal magnetism. They are enthusiastic beyond the ordinary . . . sociable . . . movable . . . a pleasure to be with. They have bright and happy dispositions. They are free from hang ups and mental blocks. These are the well adjusted people who enjoy a more fulfilling, healthy, happy life.

What is their secret? How do they live at a superior rate of high vibration? The answer is really very simple. Such people consume large amounts of oxygen. They breathe deeply and fully, utilizing every square inch of their lung capacity.

The more oxygen you can breathe into your lungs, the more energy you will have . . . the higher will be your rate of vibration. It is very much like a fire in an open fireplace . . . the more oxygen the fire gets, the brighter it will burn . . . the less it gets, the less fire and more unwanted smoke it makes.

INCREASE ENERGY WITH SUPER POWER DEEP BREATHING

At age 16, my father, Paul C. Bragg, was officially diagnosed with a *hopeless* case of tuberculosis . . . but by age 18 he had become a successful athlete. During those two years he was introduced to and cured by the Science of Natural Living – to which he dedicated the rest of his life to share with others.

Paul C. Bragg became a great-great-grandfather, to his credit . . . and in any competition requiring energy and stamina, he could outlast most people half and even less than half his age. He could type for hours without mental or physical fatigue. He enjoyed all sports. He hiked, jogged, biked, swam, lifted weights and climbed some of the world's highest mountains and he loved tennis, polo and surfing.

He kept himself in a high rate of mental and physical vibration by supplying his body with the correct fuel: natural, healthy live foods and above all, super power oxygen.

He helped people in all walks of life – musicians, singers, writers, artists, doctors, lawyers, as well as athletes and active sportsmen, office workers and housewives – to achieve the enjoyment of a superior state of healthy living.

The basic source of super-oxygen-vibration is knowing how to deeply fill your lungs with oxygen. Everyone is born with this capacity, but only a few people retain it naturally.

Whatever your age, it is never too early or too late to learn how to increase your energy by the Bragg System of Super Power Breathing. Within *months* of faithfully following the breathing exercises in this book, you too can learn how to fill your lungs with super power, energy-producing oxygen. You will enjoy the thrill of this great natural stimulation. It is far more potent than that of any artificial stimulant such as alcohol, coffee, tea, cola drinks or drugs and has no adverse side effects! In fact, the *side effects* of oxygen stimulation add up to the bonus of a longer, healthier and fuller lifetime.

LIVING AT A MEDIUM SO-SO RATE OF VIBRATION

Certain levels of vitality and energy, both mental and physical, are attained by people who live at a medium rate of vibration. While they have a fine capacity for work and play, they are not capable of the sustained effort achieved by those at a high level. Medium-vibration people tire more easily. They lack endurance, particularly under stress. Exhaustion induced by tension and strain forces them to stop and rest.

Such people simply do not get enough vital oxygen to give them that extra something to keep going under physical, mental or emotional pressures. Under extreme pressure they *run out of gas* . . . they are lacking the high vibration (deep power breathing) it takes to make the additional effort.

Why? Because they are not using the full capacity of their lungs for energy-producing oxygen . . . they can't get their *second wind*. That is the difference between the person who lives in the super, high vibration and those who have achieved only a medium rate of vibration.

MIRACLE VALUES OF THE SECOND WIND

At a high rate of vibration, when you consume your full quota of oxygen, you are able to get your *second wind* . . . and feel stronger than when you began your effort. That *second wind* is what makes the great athlete, the great politician, the great statesman, the great professional man or woman, the writer, the great singer, actor, dancer, or the go-getter.

When you learn to use the full capacity of your lungs through the Bragg System of Super Power Breathing, you will experience this wonderful stimulation of the *second wind*. Just when you think you have run out of energy and

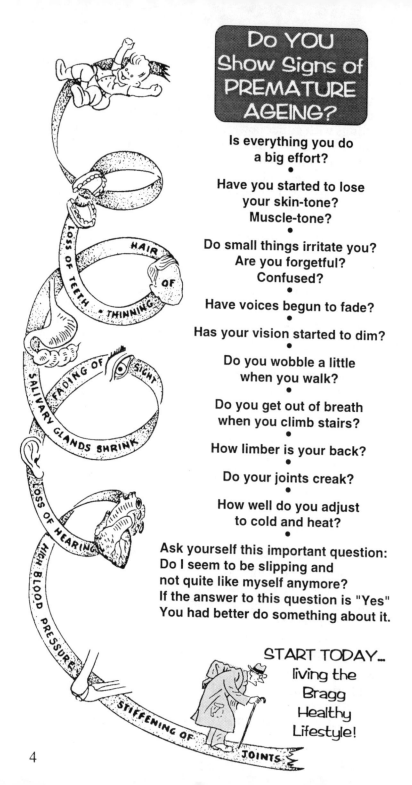

Do YOU Show Signs of PREMATURE AGEING?

Is everything you do
a big effort?

•

Have you started to lose
your skin-tone?
Muscle-tone?

•

Do small things irritate you?
Are you forgetful?
Confused?

•

Have voices begun to fade?

•

Has your vision started to dim?

•

Do you wobble a little
when you walk?

•

Do you get out of breath
when you climb stairs?

•

How limber is your back?

•

Do your joints creak?

•

How well do you adjust
to cold and heat?

•

Ask yourself this important question:
Do I seem to be slipping and
not quite like myself anymore?
If the answer to this question is "Yes"
You had better do something about it.

START TODAY...
living the
Bragg
Healthy
Lifestyle!

LOSS OF TEETH • THINNING

HAIR OF

FADING OF SIGHT

SALIVARY GLANDS SHRINK

LOSS OF HEARING

HIGH BLOOD PRESSURE

STIFFENING OF JOINTS

4

vitality . . . this sudden renewal of strength occurs. It is an experience truly difficult to describe. When you feel that you cannot take another step, that your brain power is all gone, your thinking befuddled. . . suddenly a great surge of energy courses through your entire body, and you feel as fresh as, and even stronger than when you started. What a tremendous sensation it is! When you breathe correctly, you experience this *amazing second wind.* Athletes win with this.

SHALLOW BREATHING CAUSES PREMATURE AGEING

Even the people who live at a medium rate of vibration are in the minority. In our civilized world today, I regret to report, most people are only half-alive . . . they merely exist at a very low rate of physical and mental vibration. This includes all ages . . . from early teens to late eighties (if they live that long).

Research has shown that, in modern civilized countries, only babies use their lungs as Nature intended. All too soon they acquire the unnatural *civilized* habit of shallow (low vibration) breathing. They use only the top part of their lungs. This shallow breathing starves your body of vital oxygen it must have to be truly alive. That is why you see so many people – from teenagers to oldsters – crowding doctors' offices, clinics, sanitariums, hospitals and convalescent homes, dragging through life, seeking artificial remedies and palliatives, laxatives, painkillers, tonics, sleeping pills and various other drugs for illusionary quick fixes.

Oxygen-starved people are usually nervous, and suffer from unnecessary worries as well as physical ills. Millions go to bed tired and wake up tired. They suffer from headaches, constipation, indigestion, muscular aches and pains, stiff joints, aching backs and aching feet, aching teeth and sore, receding gums, poor eyesight, poor hearing, loss of memory, sore throats and respiratory ailments such as bronchitis, asthma, sinus infections and emphysema.

These miseries and the loss of healthy bodily functions attributed to *ageing,* plague these people early in life and take them to an early grave. They suffer and die needlessly –simply because they don't know how to live a healthy lifestyle and breathe correctly! It seems incredible – but it's true.

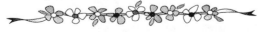

Health and intellect are two blessings of life. – Monostikoi

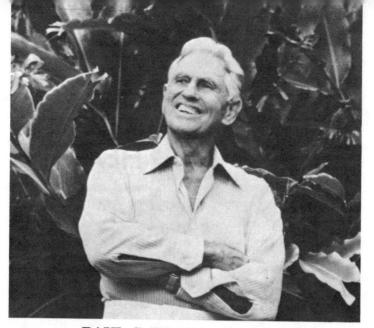

PAUL C. BRAGG, N.D., Ph.D.
World's Leading Healthy Lifestyle Authority

Paul C. Bragg's daughter Patricia and their wonderful, healthy members of the Bragg "Longer Life, Health and Happiness Club" exercise daily at the beautiful Fort DeRussy lawn, at the world famous Waikiki Beach in Honolulu, Hawaii. Membership is free and open to everyone who wishes to attend any morning - Monday through Saturday, from 9 to 10:30 am for Bragg Deep Breathing exercises and exercises for health and fitness. Often on Saturday there are health lectures on how to live a long, healthy life! The group averages 75 to 125 per day, according to the seasons. From December to March it can go up to 200. Its dedicated leaders have been carrying on the class for over 24 years. Thousands have visited the club from around the world and carried the Bragg health and fitness message to friends and relatives back home. Patricia extends an invitation to you and your friends to join the club for wholesome, healthy fellowship... when you visit Honolulu, Hawaii. Be sure also to visit the outer Hawaiian Islands (Maui, Kauai, Hawaii, and Molokai) for a fulfilling, healthy vacation.

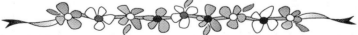

To maintain good health the body must be exercised properly (stretching, brisk walking, biking, swimming, deep breathing, good posture, etc.) and nourished wisely (natural foods), to maintain a normal weight and increase the good life of radiant health, joy and happiness. – Paul C. Bragg

6

Chapter 2

Oxygen Starvation

Suppose you are very hungry, and sit down to enjoy a well planned, nourishing meal . . . but as soon as you have eaten only one-fourth of the food, someone snatches it away and tells you that you can't have any more. What would you think of the food-snatcher?

Yet this is exactly what you do to yourself when you breathe as most people do, using only one-fourth to one-third of your lung capacity. You are starving your body much more than if you deprive it of food. You are robbing your body of its most vital, invisible nourishment – oxygen.

Without sufficient oxygen, your body cannot properly utilize the food you eat and drink, no matter how basically nourishing the food may be. Oxygen is essential to the ionization process, the breaking up of food molecules into nutrients suitable for the body's vital needs.

With an insufficient supply of oxygen, your bloodstream becomes saturated with poisonous carbon dioxide and other toxic wastes and transports these toxins throughout your body (collecting more en route), thereby suffocating your cells, instead of rejuvenating them with life-giving oxygen.

Your brain, which requires three times more oxygen than the rest of your body, suffers first. Philip Rice, M.D. states:

55% of the delinquent behavior in minors can be attributed to oxygen starvation.

Dr. Rice has worked his entire life with delinquent children.

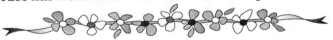

Perhaps the most valuable result of all education is the ability to make yourself do the thing you have to do, when it ought to be done, as it ought to be done, whether you like it or not!

Oxygen is the vital, precious, invisible staff of life. – Paul C Bragg

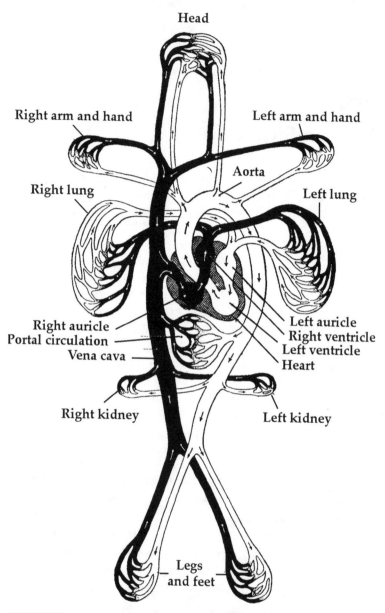

Head

Right arm and hand

Left arm and hand

Aorta

Right lung

Left lung

Right auricle
Portal circulation
Vena cava

Left auricle
Right ventricle
Left ventricle
Heart

Right kidney

Left kidney

Legs
and feet

THE HEART AND BLOOD-VESSEL SYSTEM. The diagram shows the vital, life-giving blood being pumped from the right side of the heart through the lungs where it picks up oxygen, to the left side of the heart, then through the system back to the right side of the heart again. All the blood from the digestive system goes through the portal veins; i.e., through the liver and continues its miracle mission your entire life!

8

Oxygen starvation is caused by shallow breathing, sedentary habits and a lack of exercise and fresh air. Educators who are alarmed about the decrease in the average I.Q. would do well to consider this factor. Tests and analyses are not brain food . . . life-giving oxygen is!

You can make a simple demonstration by lighting two candles and placing them side by side, a few inches apart. Now partially cover one candle with a glass . . . watch how much smaller and paler this flame becomes. If you cover the candle completely with the glass, the flame will go out in a few seconds. That is what happens in your body when you deprive it of life-giving oxygen, the invisible staff of life.

OXYGEN POWERS THE HUMAN MACHINE

The human body is a marvelous and intricate mechanism for the production of mental and physical energy. Oxygen is this mechanism's power source. Your body begins to function with your first breath and continues until your last. How well it functions depends on how well you supply it with oxygen power.

As in any heat or combustion engine, **oxygen is essential to the production of energy in your body.** Every flame consists of the union of oxygen with other elements. The gasoline that fuels your car, the natural gas or coal in a heater or furnace, the wood in a fireplace or stove all contain latent energy . . . but it cannot be released to produce heat or power until its elements are broken down and united with oxygen.

In the human body this process is called metabolism. The food you eat contains latent energy, but it is of absolutely no use to you without oxygen. To determine the general health of our bodies, we can test the rate of our basal metabolism. A laboratory determines this rate by measuring the oxygen we utilize while our body is in a resting state.

As long as you live, the body mechanism operates continuously. Even when you are asleep, your lungs and heart, your kidneys, liver and other major organs, your circulatory and nervous systems must continue to function. The amount of energy you need depends, of course, upon your activities, mental as well as physical. **The release of the energy you need depends upon your intake of oxygen and your general well-being.**

9

OXYGEN CARRIED BY THE BLOODSTREAM

Every one of the 40 trillion cells in your body demands a continuous flow of life-giving oxygen in order to stay alive, do its job, and remain healthy. This oxygen supply is carried in your bloodstream by the red blood cells, or red corpuscles . . . and there are millions of these red cells in every drop of blood.

The blood circulates in a network of 100,000 miles of blood vessels that reach every cell in the body, from those of the heart itself, to the top of the scalp and the tips of the fingers and toes. In the average individual there are about five quarts of blood circulating in this vast network.

During rest or inactivity the blood makes one round trip per minute. During activity or exercise, however, it may make as many as eight or nine round trips per minute in order to supply the necessary fuel and oxygen for increased energy, and to remove the toxins and burnt-out wastes.

The blood vessels that carry blood from the heart are known as arteries. Those that return blood to the heart are veins. Both vary greatly in size, just like streams, brooks and creeks which flow into a river, which then joins a larger river.

The smallest of both the arteries and the veins are called capillaries. They are so tiny that most are visible only under a microscope. Through these capillaries the last of the food and oxygen is given off and the transfer is made into the veins, which carry the oxygen-depleted blood and toxic wastes back to the heart for purification. Enroute to the heart most of the water-soluble wastes are transferred to the kidneys for elimination from the body through the urine. The poisonous carbon dioxide gas, a major residue of energizing oxidation, is brought back to the heart to be expelled through the lungs.

Blood is the river of life that flows through the human body. We cannot live without it. The heart pumps blood to all our body cells, supplying them with oxygen and food.

Breathing deeply, fully and completely energizes the body, calms the nerves, fills you with peace and helps keep you youthful.
– Paul C. Bragg

Most men employ the first part of life to make the rest miserable.
– La Bruyere

SUPER BREATHING DETOXIFIES & PURIFIES YOUR BLOOD

The carbon dioxide collected from all parts of the body gives the blood a bluish color when it is returned through the veins to the heart. There it enters the right auricle, the heart's upper chamber. After the auricle fills with blood, the valve into the right ventricle (lower chamber) opens, allowing the blood to pass into the ventricle. When the valve closes, the ventricle's strong muscles contract, sending blood to the lungs.

As blood travels through the capillary network in the lung sacs, it discharges its load of carbon dioxide and turns a healthy, bright red again as it absorbs the life-giving oxygen, and immediately returns to the left auricle of the heart. From there it goes into the left ventricle by similar valve action, and is pumped vigorously into the body's largest artery, the aorta. Leaving the aorta, blood travels throughout the body through a vast arterial network – taking its life-giving oxygen and nutrients to every cell of the entire body to keep you healthy.

It is the shorter or *lesser* circulation, as it is called . . . from the heart to the lungs and back . . . that is so vital to detoxify and purify the bloodstream. If the lungs are only partially filled with air, only part of the bloodstream can be cleansed. The blood which passes through the capillaries of empty air sacs cannot get rid of its carbon dioxide wastes and cannot pick up oxygen. So, instead of carrying a full quota of life-giving oxygen back to the cells of the body, the bloodstream returns with a mixture of fresh oxygen and a residue of toxic poisons. As this sluggish process continues, the proportion of carbon dioxide buildup increases causing health problems.

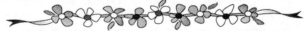

FILL YOUR LUNGS WITH SUPER, LIFE-GIVING OXYGEN

Breath Expansion Test: *before you begin your Bragg Super Power Breathing Program perform this simple test. Exhale fully and measure your deflated chest with a tape measure. Take a deep breath and measure again. After a month of practicing these exercises, take this test again. You will be amazed by how much more super, life-giving oxygen fills your lungs when you practice Bragg Super Breathing.*

YOUR AMAZING HARD-WORKING LUNGS ARE MIRACLE WORKERS

. . . for your well-being – treat them kindly! The surface area of one human lung is equal to a tennis court. On an average day your lungs move enough air in and out to fill a medium-sized room or blow up several thousand party balloons.

SHALLOW BREATHERS POISON THEMSELVES

When your breathing is shallow, you do not change the air at the base of your lungs, where two-thirds of the lung capacity is located. When you return impure blood to your body, the ill effects are seriously compounded because the blood cannot perform properly.

It is difficult for blood that is loaded with poisonous wastes to transport the relatively small amount of oxygen which it does absorb. And, it is even harder for it to carry the necessary nourishment from food. Without an adequate oxygen supply, the breaking down of food molecules into digestible elements is impaired and all bodily functions are slowed down. See why deep breathing is important for health!

With wrong diet and shallow breathing the organs of elimination are overworked . . . and underfed! But the accumulating wastes must go somewhere. Some are discharged into the sweat glands. This toxic overload produces unpleasant body odors. Other toxic wastes are deposited as heavy mucous in the sinus cavities, lungs and bronchial tubes . . . along the passages of the ears, eyes, nose and throat . . . and along the digestive tract. Hardened wastes are deposited in the movable joints and spine, where pressure on nerves sounds the warning signals of pain. Pain is Nature's red flashing alarm that something is seriously wrong with your body. Warning pain should be respected with corrective health measures right away . . . not silenced by pain-stopping drugs with their unknown side effects.

By robbing their bodies of vital oxygen, shallow breathers are actually poisoning themselves. This is auto-intoxication – or self-poisoning – for they are slowly suffocating, dying in their own body wastes and poisons. This is pneumonia – in which your body and lungs drown in their own toxins and mucus!

If someone else deliberately tried to force you to kill yourself by taking short, shallow breathes, what would you do? You'd fight back, wouldn't you? In defiance, you would breathe deeply and fully . . . cleansing your blood . . purifying your entire system . . . making your body tingle with more life and super energy, for more vital health!.

Start Practicing Bragg Super Power Breathing now!

Chapter 3

The Way You Breathe
Is The Way You Live

When You Breathe Deep and Full
You Live More Deeply and Fully

When a generous flow of oxygen is being pumped into your body, every cell becomes more alive! This enables the four main *motors* of the body . . . the heart, the lungs, the liver and the kidneys . . . to operate and perform better. Your miracle-working bloodstream purifies itself, cleanses every part of the body, eliminates the toxic wastes as Nature planned and carries fuel (food) and vital oxygen to every cell in your body.

With ample oxygen your muscles, tendons and joints function more smoothly. Your flesh becomes firmer and resilient . . . your skin clear and glowing . . . your hair lustrous. You radiate with greater health and well-being.

With deep power breathing your brain becomes more alert and your nervous system functions more perfectly. You become more free from tension and strain . . .because you can easily withstand the stresses and pressures of daily living.

Your emotions are under your control. You feel joyous and exuberant. When negative emotions try to intrude . . . such as anger, hate, jealousy, greed or fear . . . they are expelled by positive thinking along with concentrated deep breathing.

The deep breather enjoys peace of mind, tranquility and serenity. In India, the Great Masters teach deep, full breathing as the first essential for higher spiritual development. You get more perfect concentration in meditation by long, slow, deep breaths. Deep breathing stimulates the higher brain cells. The person who breathes deeply and fully thinks more clearly. Oxygen stimulates logic and intelligence. The more

Freedom and progress rest in man's continual search for truth.
Truth is the summit of being. – Ralph Waldo Emerson

THE LOWER RESPIRATORY SYSTEM

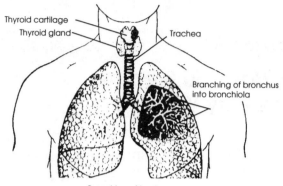

Thyroid cartilage
Thyroid gland
Trachea
Branching of bronchus into bronchiola

Branching of trachea into right and left bronchi

PATH OF BREATH

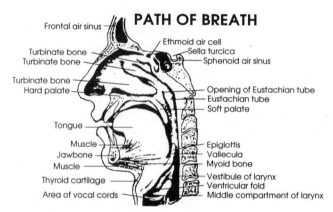

Frontal air sinus
Turbinate bone
Turbinate bone
Turbinate bone
Hard palate
Tongue
Muscle
Jawbone
Muscle
Thyroid cartilage
Area of vocal cords

Ethmoid air cell
Sella turcica
Sphenoid air sinus
Opening of Eustachian tube
Eustachian tube
Soft palate
Epiglottis
Vallecula
Myoid bone
Vestibule of larynx
Ventricular fold
Middle compartment of larynx

MECHANICS OF BREATHING

The mechanics of breathing showing the position of the diaphragm and ribs at expiration and at inspiration.

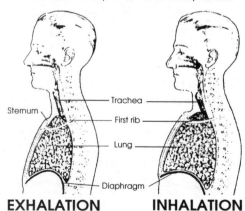

Sternum
Trachea
First rib
Lung
Diaphragm

EXHALATION   **INHALATION**

deeply and fully you breathe, the greater is your power of concentration . . . and the more fully your creative power will assert itself. You also develop greater extrasensory perception within your body. You are fine tuning your body.

Master your body. **Deep, full, super power breathing will constantly rejuvenate you to a higher vibration of living.** The more fully and deeply you breathe, the further you will travel to higher levels on the physical, mental and spiritual planes. **Start thinking now about breathing!**

GIVE THANKS TO YOUR MIRACLE-WORKING LUNGS

Every living thing breathes. Plants breathe through pores in their leaves. In the marvelous balance of Nature, plants breathe in carbon dioxide and give off vital oxygen . . . while animals inhale oxygen and exhale carbon dioxide. In a healthy natural balance, both thrive! But people have played havoc with this natural balance by destroying forests and covering grass with pavement. They continue to add pollutants from motorized traffic and industry to air that is already over-polluted with an excess of carbon dioxide. Wildlife, which has survived slaughter by man, suffocates in such polluted air. Fish die in polluted waters. How long can people survive in the midst of the environmental poisons which they continually create? This is a question of concern. Read the classic book, *Silent Spring* by Rachel Carson, available in most libraries. If followed, her wise advice would have saved America billions of dollars by now! We need more Carsons today!

Every animal extracts oxygen from the environment in which it lives. Through their gills, fish extract oxygen from water (H_2O). Insects get it from the air through alveoli or air cells in individual openings set in segments of their bodies. Worms and other invertebrates breathe through their skin pores.

Vertebrate animals, and the human race, have that wonderful mechanism: the lungs. The mechanical equivalent would be a pair of bellows. Lungs are far more intricate and adaptable.

Composed of spongy, porous tissue, the lungs are a pair of conical shaped organs which, with the heart in the center, occupy the thoracic cavity or chest – the upper half of the human torso – and are protected by the amazing and protective rib cage. The apex of each lung reaches just above the collar bone; the base extends to the waistline.

The lungs are composed of some 800 million *alveoli* – air cells or sacs of elastic tissue – which can expand or contract like tiny balloons. If these little air sacs were flattened out and laid side by side, the flattened alveoli would cover an area of 100 square yards.

Tiny capillaries (blood vessels) thread the elastic walls of each of the millions of air sacs . . . and it is through these that the blood passes to discharge its load of poisonous carbon dioxide and absorb the vital, life-giving oxygen. The average person has five to six quarts of blood which must be cleansed continually.

Air inhaled through the nose and mouth reaches the alveoli through an intricate system of tubes, beginning with the large trachea, or windpipe, which is kept rigid by rings of cartilage in its walls. The trachea extends through the neck into the chest, where it divides into two branches, or bronchi, one leading into each lung. The bronchi divide into a number of successively smaller branches to reach every air sac.

Each lung is enveloped in a protective elastic membrane, the pleura, whose inner layer is attached to the lung and whose outer layer forms the lining of the thoracic cavity inside the rib cage. One end of each rib is attached to the spinal column, but the front of the rib cage is open. This allows the lungs to expand and contract.

When you breathe deeply, filling every air sac, your thoracic cavity expands as your lungs fill to capacity with six to ten pints of air (which varies according to body build and size), and occupy between 200 to over 300 cubic inches. This marvelous breathing mechanism is yours for free! You are born with it. It functions without conscious effort, yet without it, you cannot exist. **Right now start slow, deep breathing.**

No human invention, however ingenious, can equal the human breathing apparatus. The *iron lung* is misnamed. Lifesaver that it is, it is merely a cumbersome contraption outside your body that replaces paralyzed muscles . . . enabling those wonderful human lungs to function.

Perhaps if human beings had to pay a fabulous price for their lungs, they would use them to full capacity all the time. Think of the price you pay for not using them? Remember, we are always *only one breath away from death!*

THE HEALTH IMPORTANCE OF CLEAN AIR

It is essential to breathe clean air. Air as free as possible from such chemicals as smog, car exhaust, natural gas appliance fumes and many other toxic chemical pollutants. The air also needs to be as free as possible from dust, dust mites and their fecal matter, mold, animal danders and pollen. In varying degrees everyone's health is helped by clean air. It is vitally important to live and work in an area which has clean air without harmful fumes and it's equally important to keep our homes pure and clean. Most people do not become well until they breathe clean air, maintain a healthy diet and live a healthy lifestyle. **Bragg Books can be your faithful health guides, by your side – night or day.**

We advise those who live in smog-ridden, polluted cities to obtain a good air filter. We especially recommend filters which contain charcoal and a high efficiency particulate air HEPA filter. The charcoal removes most of the chemicals and the HEPA filter removes most of the particles. To be effective in an average sized room the flow rate through the filter should be over two hundred cubic feet of air per minute. The wise driver will also install an activated charcoal filter in his car for cleaning the air while driving in air polluted cities

For information on the best room and car air filters call 1-800-446-1990 or send an SASE to: PURE AIR 7340 Hollister Avenue, Goleta, California 93117

When we are born, our lungs are shiny and new, fresh and clean, rosy in color. If we could live in a dust-free atmosphere and breathe correctly all our lives, our lungs would remain *as good as new* throughout a lifetime of use.

But what most lungs get is abuse, Some of this comes from external causes. The lungs are the only organs of the body which are directly affected by conditions external to it, specifically, the air we breathe!

Nature has provided protection against a normal amount of dust contamination – tiny hairs in the nose to serve as filters and with moist mucous in the passages leading to the lungs to trap dust particles which we then expel through the nose or mouth.

Breathing is the greatest pleasure in life. — Papini

The tonsils also serve as guards to trap germs. The lungs protect themselves remarkably well by expelling carbon dioxide through oxygenation and by discharging toxins into the blood for elimination via the kidneys.

However, most civilized people today live in very unnatural conditions. Certainly there are an abnormal amount of pollutants in the air we breathe, especially in urban areas. Our lungs are often overloaded with more contaminants than they can handle, and these are passed along into the bloodstream and to other parts of the body. The lungs of a modern city dweller become brownish from oil smog, and even in farming country, the lungs must contend with excess dust, poisonous pesticides, sprays and chemicals.

A recent study in California showed that 275 people a year died in two counties east of Los Angeles as a result of the particulates in smog. They estimated that the total number of overall smog related deaths in the two smog riddled counties could be as high as 545 people annually.

WHAT SMOKING DOES TO YOUR LUNGS

With all these nearly inescapable health hazards to overcome, it seems incredible that anyone would deliberately inhale smoke into their lungs endangering their health!!!

Nicotine is poison. **It immediately effects lung function and constricts your cardiovascular system. It destroys Vitamin C, which is vital to your health and immune system. In 12 hours of not smoking nicotine blood levels fall, heart and lungs begin healing, if you smoke, stop now!**

The air sacs are further damaged by tobacco tars and carbon particles that lodge in the walls of these important balloon-like cells . . . causing them to lose their elasticity . . . and ultimately breaking them down altogether. The result? **Emphysema** – the killer disease where destruction of the air sacs function slowly smothers its victim from within.

Of the 50 million smoking Americans 1/3 to 1/2 will die from smoke-related diseases. Smoking creates a desire for caffeine and sugar and twice as many smokers drink alcohol compared to nonsmokers. Clinical evidence proves that smokers have a far greater incidence of cancer of the lungs, larynx, pharynx, esophagus, mouth, colon, rectum and breast.

Smoking introduces two deadly poisons into the body: *arsenic* **and** *carbon monoxide.* Of course, if you insist on committing suicide by smoking, no one can stop you. If you really want to save your lungs, your health and your life, you can succeed through persistence and strong will. It may not happen the first time you try to quit, but the attempt is a good sign, a positive step towards 100% healthy living.

In our Bragg Health Crusade Lectures throughout the world, we have had health students in our classes who have smoked for as long as 50 years. They decided to stop smoking and succeeded. So can you! (Smokers should read about the deadly effect of smoking on the heart in our book, *How to Keep the Heart Healthy and Fit.* (See back pages for Bragg Book info.)

Here's a tip from a writer friend of mine, who over the years had acquired the habit of lighting a cigarette whenever she paused to correlate the next sequence of thought. She said, *when it dawned on me what I was doing, I felt like a complete fool. – I stopped smoking! It was destroying my health. Now, instead of a cigarette, I take a full, deep breath and I'm healthier, my thoughts come faster and more clearly than ever.*

She finally realized that she did this because her brain was calling for more oxygen and what she actually needed and wanted was a deep breath – but she was inhaling smoke instead of oxygen, thus defeating her purpose. Instead of being refreshed, she became more tired and started ageing.

If you are a smoker – try this! When you reach for a cigarette (or cigar or pipe) . . . stop! Take a long, slow deep breath, filling every air sac in your lungs . . . hold it, while your red blood cells become re-oxygenated . . . then exhale slowly and completely, emptying every bit of poisonous carbon dioxide from your lungs. You will feel a new surge of energy from the top of your scalp to the soles of your feet . . . a relaxing and incredibly rejuvenating sensation which you can never get from using tobacco or any other artificial stimulants! The surest way to quit a bad habit is to replace it with a good one. The greatest benefit to your life and health would be to replace smoking with deep breathing!

LOOK AT THE SICK AND DYING PEOPLE.
– John Thomas, author of *Young Again, How to Reverse Aging*

SMOKING FACTS ARE SHOCKING AND DEADLY!

✞ Tobacco will eventually kill just over 1/5 of all the people now living in the developed world – approx. 250 million.

✞ Of the 50 million smoking Americans 1/3 to 1/2 will die from smoke related disease and reduce their life expectancy by 9 years on average.

✞ Smoking acts as both a stimulant and a depressant, depending upon the smoker's emotional state.

✞ The average pack-a-day smoker takes about 70,000 *hits* of nicotine each year.

✞ "Secondhand smoke" hurts nonsmokers: it speeds up their heart rate, raises their blood pressure and doubles the amount of toxic carbon monoxide in their blood.

✞ Secondary smoke contains more nicotine, tar and cadmium (leading to hypertension, bronchitis and emphysema) than mainstream smoke.

✞ The children of smokers are born with lower body weight and smaller lungs and greater health problems.

✞ Lung illnesses are twice as common in smoker's children.

✞ Children and teenagers make up 90% of the new smokers in the United States – and teenage smoking is on the rise.

✞ Tobacco is the main introduction to more deadly drugs.

✞ Teens who smoke are far more likely to engage in other risky and life-threatening behaviors than nonsmoking teenagers, including using other dangerous drugs, violence, gangs, carrying weapons and engaging in premarital sexual activity which often result in pregnancy or even disease.

THE COMMON COLD IS THE BODY'S CLEANSING PROCESS

Any day in winter over 30 million Americans are suffering with *a bad cold*. Adults average five to six colds per season, children and teenagers often get between six and twelve.

Are these colds necessary? How do people *catch cold*? What causes the common cold? Medical science has learned how to control many diseases that are far more serious, but remains baffled by the common cold. Is the culprit an unfilterable virus, as has been suggested? Is it brought on by sitting in a draft, getting chilled, getting one's feet wet?

There are many beliefs. But there seems to be only one sure fact – people who are in perfect health don't *catch colds*. My dad spent a year living in the Arctic country among the Eskimos. He never had a cold, and neither did they. He had the same experience in the South Seas, in the Balkans, among the nomads of the Middle East and with the primitive tribes of Africa. The common factor among all these people is that they breathe pure air, eat simple, natural foods, and get plenty of exercise and sleep. By following this same basic regimen, my Dad remained free of colds even in the midst of civilization.

Based on his research, he believed that the *common cold* is Nature's method of detoxifying the body. Most people are shallow breathers who exist on civilization's average, devitalized foods. A cesspool of toxins starts accumulating and clogging their bodies. It's important to live healthy!

When these accumulated poisons reach a point beyond the toxic tolerance of the body, the natural vital forces of the body set up a healing crisis. A rise in body temperature, or fever, is induced to burn up many toxic poisons . . . while others are eliminated by a heavy discharge of mucous from the nose, mouth and throat. If the toxic overload is very heavy, there may also be a discharge of mucous from the bowels and also some diarrhea.

Instead of being alarmed, be grateful that your natural vital forces are strong enough to take command and get rid of the toxic trash that you have accumulated. Don't try to block this natural healing process with drugs. Work with Nature. Rest and fast. Drink fruit and vegetable juices or herb teas and distilled water . . . but take nothing else into your stomach during this crisis period. Breathe deeply and fully to supply your body with that great purifier, oxygen.

Your body is a self-healing and self-repairing miracle . . . and will fight for its life against a great deal of abuse. When you follow Nature's Laws . . . and live a healthy lifestyle as we do, you can have a painless, tireless, ageless body, as we have.

If you *catch cold*, remember you are passing through a natural cleansing healing crisis . . . and heed the warning. Mother Nature is telling you: *You have allowed your body to become poisoned with toxic wastes. Work with me now to cleanse your system of these poisons . . . and once this cleansing crisis is passed, continue to work and keep your body clean by following my Natural Living Laws.*

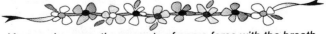

You can increase the currents of nerve force with the breath, and send it to heal parts of your body. – Yogi Ramacharaka

OXYGEN: THE VITAL SOURCE OF GOOD HEALTH

Often people tell me that they have a bad case of the *flu*. When I ask where they got it, I usually hear that old broken record, *You know, the flu's going around. Everyone's got it.* I ask, *Where can I find it? I'd like to meet some flu germs.* They stare at me in utter amazement.

To help them out of their mental confusion, I then explain that when you live a healthy lifestyle on a diet of natural foods – foods free from all refining, processing and chemical additives – and breathe fully and deeply, you build a powerful immunity against germs that cause harmful viruses.

No germ, for example, can live in pure, freshly squeezed orange juice, because there is nothing in pure orange juice for it to feed on. All germs, regardless of their names, are scavengers. They feed on decaying matter.

It's our personal opinion, based on experience and research, that a 100% healthy natural foods diet – in combination with the enormous amount of pure oxygen pumped into the body by the vigorous breathing exercises taught in this book – provides a natural immunity against infectious diseases. Oxygen is the powerful, invisible staff of life.

Oxygen is the great purifier and natural cleanser. Oxygen is not only the energizing factor which makes it possible for the body to eliminate the putrefactive matter on which germs thrive . . . it also exterminates the germs themselves. As you pump more oxygen into your body, the greater ability you give your body to ward off germs and infections!

When we practice Super Power Breathing, we increase our cardiovascular respiratory power. We purify and energize our bloodstream to carry purifying, vitalizing oxygen to the heart and throughout the entire cardiovascular system.

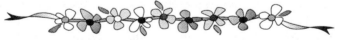

Deep breathing increases healing currents of Nerve Force and sends it throughout the body. – Patricia Bragg

Nerve Force contains much of its power in the breath. –Yoga Sutras

Viruses and microbes (such as flu, colds, AIDS, arterial plaque and cancer cells) live best in low oxygen environments. They are anaerobic. That means increase the oxygen level around them, and they die. –Ed McCabe

Chapter 4

Your Diaphragm

THE KEY TO BRAGG SUPER POWER BREATHING

What is the secret of deep super power breathing? How do you draw in air to the very base of your lungs? Certainly not by merely sniffing it in through your nose nor by gasping it in through your mouth.

Babies breathe naturally by using their diaphragms to create suction which pulls air into the lungs. Air may enter the body through either the nose or the mouth, but the force which draws it in to fill the air sacs of the lungs to capacity comes from the muscular action of the diaphragm.

The diaphragm is a dome-shaped sheet of strong muscle fibers that separates the thoracic (upper) half of your body containing the heart and lungs, from the abdominal (lower) cavity which houses the organs of digestion and elimination. The diaphragm stretches from the sternum (breastbone) in front across the bottom of the ribs to the backbone.

As the diaphragm expands and flattens moving downward, it produces suction within the chest cavity, pulling air into the lungs (inhalation). When the diaphragm relaxes and rises, it forces air out of the lungs (exhalation). Both operations are equally important: inhalation to bring in life-giving oxygen; exhalation to expel every bit of poisonous carbon dioxide.

AROMATHERAPY

Aroma has the power to work miracles, to uplift and heal. Essential oils can help improve physical and emotional health. Treat yourself to the delights and fragrances of essential oils. Also smelling roses, flowers and fruit blossoms is recharging. You will enjoy a wonderful experience and enhance your health.

CHEST VERSUS DIAPHRAGMATIC BREATHING

Chest breathing is breathing resulting from the movement of the rib section of the trunk, especially the upper section of the chest. When a person inhales, the chest expands, becoming larger. When he exhales, the chest relaxes, becoming smaller. When performed to the limit of inhalation and exhalation, this is an excellent form of internal exercise. It develops the chest and has many health benefits.

A great deal is made about *chest expansion* . . . the number of inches which the chest expands from a relaxed position (after exhalation) to that when the lungs are filled with air. However, people with large chests are not any better off than people with average-sized chests who use their breathing organs efficiently to spread oxygen throughout their bodies.

Chest breathing is naturally employed by the body only during strenuous exertion. It might be termed a form of *forced breathing.* It is an emergency measure. Unfortunately, most people rob themselves of oxygen when they breathe using only a minimum of the top of the chest.

Diaphragmatic breathing is the natural method for which the human body was designed. When the diaphragm expands, it not only expands the chest cavity and draws air into the lungs, it also expands the abdominal cavity. This doesn't draw in air; it stretches the abdominal muscles and organs. When the diaphragm relaxes, it not only expels air from the lungs and further exercises the rib muscles, but it also tones and tightens the abdominal muscles.

INTERNAL MASSAGE BY DIAPHRAGMATIC ACTION

The diaphragm's expansion and relaxation on the muscles and organs of the abdomen is highly beneficial. To combat the pull of gravity and hold the abdominal organs in place, our abdominal muscles need all the exercise we can give them. Correct, natural diaphragmatic breathing, along with daily exercise and good posture helps accomplishes this.

Diaphragmatic action also provides important massage for the heart and chest, stomach area, liver, intestines, kidneys, gallbladder, spleen and pancreas, stimulating blood circulation and aiding these organs to perform the functions which are essential to maintaining our life and health.

The dual action of the diaphragm, which affects the upper thoracic organs (heart and lungs) and the lower abdominal organs, is a vital factor in good blood circulation. Especially as blood returns through the veins to the heart. The forceful pumping thrust of the heart muscles sends blood coursing through the arteries. This force is almost spent by the time the bloodstream has dispensed oxygen, nutrients and collected wastes, and is ready to return to the heart through the veins. The return trip is dependent upon the contraction of the muscles and muscular walls of the viscera (the internal organs of the body, especially those contained within the abdominal and thoracic cavities), which push the blood through valves set in the veins to guide the bloodstream back to the heart. The rhythmic massage of the abdominal organs by the respiratory muscles plays a vital role in this vital venous circulation.

Diaphragmatic breathing also stimulates *peristalsis,* the rhythmic, wavelike motion of the intestines, which promotes digestion and the elimination of solid and semisolid toxic wastes. Changing from chest to diaphragmatic breathing has helped thousands to correct chronic constipation, gas, heartburn, indigestion and liver troubles, etc.

BRAGG SUPER POWER BREATHING CALMS THE NERVES

The *solar plexus,* the *powerhouse* of the body – a network of ganglia (independent groups of nerve cells) and nerves which control every important vital organ in the abdominal cavity – is located in the very center of the diaphragm. The more stimulation you give the diaphragm, the more circulation the solar plexus receives and the greater the nerve energy going to your vital organs. The important *pneumo-gastric nerve (pneumo,* lungs; *gastro,* stomach) passes through the diaphragm and also benefits from diaphragmatic action.

Open your mind for the doors of wisdom are never shut.
– Ben Franklin

Breathing only in the upper chest avoids the strong creative energies of the abdomen and sexual organs. Breathing only in the abdomen avoids the powerfully creative energies of the heart and throat. – Michael G. White

Diaphragmatic breathing has a tranquilizing rhythm, stimulates circulation and generally rejuvenates the body. These factors have a calming effect upon the entire nervous system. Diaphragmatic breathing breaks up the paralyzing nerve tension so often observed in people with supersensitive or jangled nerves. For more details about the beneficial effects of deep breathing on the nerves, read our book, *Building a Powerful Nerve Force.* (See back pages for book info.)

Yoga teaches that deep, rhythmic breathing attunes one to the *rhythm of the universe* . . . in other words, one lives in rhythmic harmony with Nature. *Prana,* the yoga word for *breath,* also means *absolute energy* or *vital cosmic energy* . . . which, according to the teachings of yoga, is stored in the solar plexus when we breathe correctly.

AYURVEDIC HEALTH AND FITNESS LIFESTYLE

Ayurveda is an ancient health system developed in India thousands of years ago which is reemerging as a important modern model of health and fitness. In the teachings of Ayurveda each person's mind-body type is determined and then specific diets, exercise and lifestyle routines are prescribed for that person.

Essential to Ayurveda is yoga, and its practice, and the importance of breathing correctly. Yoga breathing helps your mind and body become one. Exercise can help you learn to maintain your composure. Learning to breathe correctly, so that you remain calm and focused during exercise, will help you remain calm in other real life stress situations.

Yoga breathing is nose breathing. It has been known for centuries to slow the heart, lower blood pressure and relieve stress. Because it is a more efficient way to get oxygen into your body, it will enhance athletic performance. To practice it, start by doing some yoga stretches. Then walk with gradually increasing speed – breathing only through your nose – until you are jogging. When you can no longer breathe comfortably, slow down until you can again breathe comfortably through your nose. Do this back and forth several times – jogging, walking, jogging, walking, always breathing through your nose. Finish with some more yoga stretches. Practiced regularly this will calm you, give you greater oxygen and increased health and vitality.

Chapter 5

The Importance of Good Posture

Humans, from skeleton to skin, are built to stand, sit and walk erect. Now that we have reviewed the way your breathing apparatus operates, you can readily understand how essential correct posture is to correct breathing. When you slump, you squeeze your lungs (and other organs) into a cramped position and seriously limit the operation of your diaphragm. You become a shallow breather, able to use only the top portion of your lungs. When you sit bent over a desk, at study or work, you rob your body of maximum oxygen, impair circulation, hamper the functions of your heart and vital organs, and scrunch your muscles and bones into unnatural positions. Then you wonder why you're so fatigued! You probably also cross your legs, further blocking the circulation, preparing the way for broken capillaries and varicose veins, backaches and headaches

It is likely that you maintain the same poor posture when on your feet: standing or walking with your shoulders and head drooping or neck upthrust. You cannot improve matters by going to the opposite extreme: distorting your body and all of its components by an exaggerated reversal, i.e., thrusting your shoulders and hips back and sucking in your stomach.

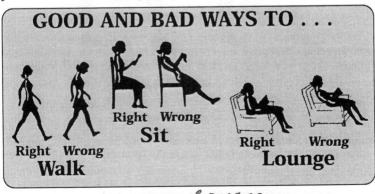

GOOD AND BAD WAYS TO . . .

Right Wrong
Sit

Right Wrong
Walk

Right Wrong
Lounge

Accuse not nature, she hath done her part; do thou but thine.
– John Milton, Paradise Lost

CORRECT HEALTHY POSTURE IMPORTANT TO HEALTH

Don't make an S of your body in either direction. For correct posture, align your body with an imaginary plumbline from the center of the top of your head through the center of your pelvis to midway between the arches of your feet.

When you sit, keep your trunk in the same position. Sit on your hips, with your feet flat on the floor or with your ankles lightly crossed. You can work for hours at your desk in this position without fatigue. But it's best to stop every hour for a good body stretch. Stand, stretch your spine up and do some front, then back shoulder rolls. Walk as often as possible, hold the same healthy posture, letting your arms swing naturally in rhythm with your stride.

WHICH POSTURE ARE YOU?

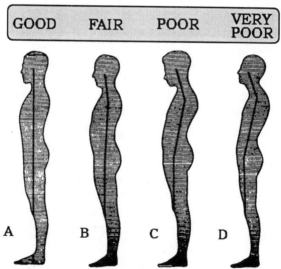

| GOOD | FAIR | POOR | VERY POOR |

A   B   C   D

(A) **GOOD: head, trunk, thigh in straight line; chest high and forward; abdomen flat; back curves normal.**

(B) **FAIR: head forward; abdomen prominent; exaggerated curve in upper back; slightly hollow back.**

(C) **POOR: relaxed (fatigue) posture; head forward; abdomen relaxed; shoulder blades prominent; hollow back.**

(D) **VERY POOR: head forward badly; very exaggerated curve in upper back; abdomen relaxed; chest flat-sloping; hollow back.**

BRAGG POSTURE EXERCISE BRINGS MIRACULOUS CHANGES

Stand with feet nine inches apart, tighten your butt and suck in your stomach muscles, lift up ribcage, stretch spine up, chest out, shoulders back, and chin up slightly. Line up straight (nose plumbline straight to belly button), drop hands to your sides and swing arms to normalize your posture. Look in the mirror – see the improvement! Do these posture exercises often – miraculous changes will happen! You are retraining and strengthening your muscles to stand straight for a healthier, more fit body and greater youthfulness. **Start practicing good posture and do this posture exercise now!**

WEAR LOOSE, COMFORTABLE CLOTHING

Now don't spoil it all with tight clothing! Restrictive clothing such as tight belts, collars, undergarments and even tight shoes can hamper breathing, blood circulation and the functioning of major organs. It can also throw your body off balance and out of alignment and can especially jangle your nerves. The sloppy dress of teenagers, worn as an outward show of rebellion against conventional uptight adult clothing, indicates an unconscious, but natural rebellion of the human body against restrictive clothing. The trend toward comfortable sports clothes and shoes (sandals) is healthier.

My father prided himself on being able to endure the coldest weather wearing only a small amount of clothing. And he swam in all parts of the world in all kinds of weather. He was known for his cold-water swimming and was welcomed as a member at Polar Bear Clubs around the world.

On several occasions, Dad and the noted Dr. Robert Jackson had great sport breaking the ice and swimming with the Boston Brownies of the famous "L" Street Bath House in Boston, Massachusetts. Here you find some of the finest physical specimens in the world, including people in their sixties, seventies, eighties and even nineties. The same is true of the Polar Bears of Coney Island and New York City, the cold water swimmers at Montrose Beach in Chicago and at Bradford Beach in Milwaukee.

All these hearty people who enjoy swimming in ice-cold water are deep and full breathers. Many of them are our health students to whom we have taught our Bragg System of Super Power Breathing. When you Super Power Breathe, you enjoy cold water swimming, because it's invigorating and energizing.

POSTURE CHART

	PERFECT	FAIR	POOR
HEAD			
SHOULDERS			
SPINE			
HIPS			
ANKLES			
NECK			
UPPER BACK			
TRUNK			
ABDOMEN			
LOWER BACK			

Your posture carries you through life from your head to your feet. Your body is your human vehicle – and is truly a miracle! Respect and protect it by living the Bragg Healthy Lifestyle for a long, fulfilled life. – Patricia Bragg

30

But I don't recommend that everyone jump into ice-cold water! Let's leave that to the people who have built a body with perfect thermostatic control. I want to give you an idea of how much power your body can develop when you are filled with oxygen at all times. There is no limit to your powers of resistance. There is no feeling of well-being as great as when every cell in the body is filled with precious life-giving oxygen!

OPERA SINGERS, BALLET DANCERS AND CHAMPION ATHLETES ARE DEEP BREATHERS

Breath control, by deep diaphragmatic breathing, is vital for all professional singers. Without benefit of loudspeakers, the voices of the early great opera singers have filled the auditoriums of the Metropolitan, La Scala and other famous opera houses throughout the world. What diaphragms they had! Look at the build of these men and women. They have beautiful, perfect posture, superior development of the torso and tremendous lung capacity. Listen to the great recorded voices of Enrico Caruso and Mario Lanza in addition to the current three tenors who are thrilling the world – Luciano Pavarotti, Placido Domingo and Jose Carreras. Hear their perfect voice control, from the softest pure note to the swell of a great crescendo.

Study the lives of these extraordinary people and you will find that they lived and are living in perfect health, filled with energy and charm, regardless of age. Most of these deep breathers live remarkably long, productive, happy lives.

The same is true of great dancers. Dad's friends, Ruth St. Dennis and Ted Shawn thrilled audiences throughout their long lifetimes, from their teens into their seventies. Deep diaphragmatic breathing was the key to the tremendous energy and muscular control demanded by their spectacular dances and also the key to their long, healthy, radiant lives.

Deep diaphragmatic breathing is a basic component to the rigorous training of all the famous ballet companies . . . as well as the great Fred Astaire/Gene Kelly type of dancers and the rollicking Rockettes of New York's Rockefeller Center – many are Bragg Health followers. In order to have super energy, most dancers find it is important to live a healthy lifestyle and most are long-lived, maintaining perpetual youthfulness.

(P.S. I've danced with Astaire, Kelly and Murray, it was thrilling! – Patricia)

The beauty, strength and endurance of North African dancers amazes me. Their secret was the excellent development of the diaphragm in breathing. As a result of its action in drawing in large quantities of fresh air, these women have exquisite skin and complexion, sparkling eyes and remarkable grace and body suppleness.

Even if you aren't a singer or dancer, there is no reason why you shouldn't enjoy good health and a long, happy life. Without having to undergo the rigorous training of a professional performer, you can profit by their key secrets: deep diaphragmatic breathing; regular exercise; a healthy lifestyle and a natural diet.

Begin with correct posture. This is essential before you can breathe correctly. Whenever you are walking, standing or sitting, always lift up the chest and diaphragm. By doing this, you will constantly be using the most important muscles in the entire body.

The key to firm body muscles is good posture. Poor posture puts your heart, lungs and all of your *working machinery* into a viselike grip which impairs circulation and efficiency. Keep saying to yourself, *I must lift up the chest and diaphragm.* In that way, you will be exercising during all of your waking hours. **Good posture brings an inner strength and tone to the muscles that no exercise can provide.**

Correct posture is vital to good health and a long life. Keep a straight line from the chin to the toes when standing. Don't slump in your chair when sitting. Keep the head, chest and diaphragm held high. It may tire you at first because most people have acquired poor posture habits. But once you give strength and tone to the many muscles which control good posture, you will find that you can maintain good posture and will be more relaxed and free from fatigue.

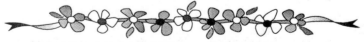

You can control your emotions — not by suppressing them —
but by learning to breathe through them.

The human body has one ability not possessed by any machine
— the ability to repair itself. — George E. Crile, Jr., M.D.

NORMALIZE YOUR FIGURE

You can actually create a fitter body and a more normal figure by correct posture and breathing exercises – no matter where you begin. All deep breathing exercises are building exercises, because oxygen is the invisible food, the life-giving force for the body and is needed by your 75 trillion cells and aids your assimilation of food. The same exercises will build up a person who is underweight, and trim down a person who is overweight. Breathing correctly is normal, and relearning correct breathing returns one to the healthy state of birth . . . and helps keep you there.

To be alive and thrill to the joy of living, you must learn to breathe correctly! You must learn to breathe with every cell of your lungs. It is then and only then that you raise your rate of physical vibration to its highest level for super energy.

You can burn off fat by internal combustion. You can help firm your flesh and keep it firm . . . normalize your figure into its naturally pleasing curves . . . by correct deep breathing habits, along with brisk walking, exercise and a healthy diet.

NO ONE CAN BREATHE FOR YOU

You can build a new figure, a new You – inside and out – vibrant, healthy, tingling with the joy of life. Remember, you and You Alone have this power. No one can breathe for you!

And this power has no value unless it is used . . . and used every day. By daily Bragg Super Power Breathing you can build perfect blood circulation. You become oxygen recharged. You will no longer feel fatigued at the least physical effort.

Breathing exercises bring sparkle to your eyes, a glow to your flesh and adds vim and vigor to your step. You will be more mentally alert. Your reflexes will function more perfectly. You will feel fit and have a sense of well-being that is a far greater treasure than any material possession.

Oxygen is the most valuable of all elements and you can have all you can breathe in for free. You have only to learn how to fully utilize it with daily Bragg Super Power Breathing. By practicing these exercises you will develop long, slow breathing at all times. The person who takes fewer, but deeper breaths per minute enjoys greater health, more endurance, more vitality and energy and a longer, more youthful life!

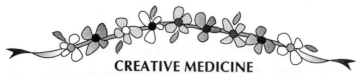

CREATIVE MEDICINE

It is no oversimplification to say that our health comes from the soil. No matter how many physicians and health professionals we train, and how much curative or preventative medicine they may practice, we cannot attain optimum health until our attention is focused on preventative medicine, and thereby learn to keep and even improve our health. To build and maintain healthy soil is the real fundamental service. Creative medicine must be founded on growing healthy organic foods. Thus alone can we create real health for our people – only through creating a sound, healthy and prosperous organic-minded agriculture.

– Dr. Jonathan Foreman, *The Land*

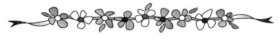

MONDAY TO JOY-DAY

There are days when you feel buried in the blues. You get up feeling depressed and pessimistic. You look worried. The world just isn't spinning in your direction, Yesterday you had it on a string, but today it has you beneath its weight.

What to do? We should realize that we are destined to have these days from time to time. They are as natural as rain. If we were always happy we'd not appreciate our joys. If we didn't have hard knocks, we wouldn't appreciate the pleasant times so much. Maybe it takes Monday morning blues to make a week well-balanced.

– Dr. P. DeWitt Fox, *Health Culture*

SLOW ME DOWN, LORD

Slow me down, Lord
Ease the pounding of my heart by the quieting of my mind.
Steady my hurried pace with a vision
        of the eternal reach of time.
Give me, amid the confusion of the day,
        the calmness of the everlasting hills.
Break the tensions of my nerves and muscles
        with the soothing music of the singing streams
        that live in my memory.
Help me to know the magical, restoring power of sleep.
Teach me the art of taking minute vacations
        – of slowing down to look at a flower, to chat with a friend,
        to pat a dog, to read a few lines from a good book.
Slow me down, Lord, and inspire me to send my roots deep
        into the soil of life's enduring values
        that I may grow toward the stars of my greater destiny.

Chapter 6

Preparing for Bragg
Super Power Breathing

The Bragg Breathing Exercises and Healthy Lifestyle slowly work with your entire body. Most humans are victims of two bad habits: shallow breathing and incorrect posture. These habits must be overcome. Muscles must be strengthened, especially the diaphragm and the abdominal muscles. Unused lung air sacs must be opened and revitalized.

Perhaps you have already experienced a *stitch in the side* when you have had to run to catch a bus or plane, or while doing some unaccustomed exercise. Actually this is a good sign, if you will profit by it. It is good to exercise to the point of getting that *stitch*. What it really means is that you have discovered a large area of unused lung cells, which have remained closed most of your life, since childhood games, that are now opening to receive the fresh air you are pumping in through your efforts to breathe deeply. The diaphragm's of older people become semi-paralyzed from non-use, but exercise and deep breathing will change that!

These unused cells are slightly stuck together and collapsed upon themselves. The sharp pain is due to the air forcing them apart. Continue to breathe deeply, even if you have caught the bus, plane or stopped your exercise. The distress will pass, your unused cells will become activated. You will have made an important step forward in deep breathing and achieving greater Super Power and Super Health.

If you experience that *stitch* during the preparatory exercises which I am going to give you, you will understand what it is and not be alarmed. Just keep on breathing!

A wise man should consider that health is the greatest of human blessings and learn how, by his own thought, to derive benefit from his illnesses. Change any unhealthy living habits to 100% healthy habits and start now!

If you don't use it, you lose it – it's true in mind, body and spirit.

FOR MORE SUPER ENERGY
PRACTICE BRAGG POSTURE EXERCISES DAILY

Correct posture allows the chest to expand so that the lungs can be filled with air. The lungs operate like millions of tiny balloons. Suction is created by the action of the diaphragm and its auxiliary muscles of the chest and abdomen. This suction fills them with air. The lungs themselves are passive and cannot breathe independently.

Remember, the lungs are attached to the walls of the rib cage by the pleural membrane. If the sternum, or breastbone, is carried high and the bony rib cage expanded, the lungs are held up in position so they can be filled with air. The uplifted diaphragm, in turn, tends to draw into position the sagging or prolapsed organs of the abdomen.

Most occupations today, however – from assembly line to desk – have a tendency to pull us down from an erect position. Many people carry the chest like a collapsed accordion, with shoulders sagging and the chest deflated, which again puts your heart and breathing apparatus in a tight, viselike grip.

To counteract this health and energy sapping tendency, a special exercise is needed. Stand with feet together. Now raise the hands high overhead, at the same time rising high on the toes. See how high you can lift up your chest . . . drawing in the abdominal muscles. Stretch up and up . . . as if trying to touch the ceiling. *Repeat this posture exercise ten times.* Also – do not try to do any special breathing. Just breathe naturally, or what is natural for you at the time.

This exercise is designed to strengthen the muscles which control the erect posture of the body. Stretching is one of the greatest tools for building health. It is the universal exercise of the animal kingdom. Wild animals are beautiful examples of natural living. House pets (cats, dogs, etc.) all stretch daily. *Always do this stretching exercise, after sitting for a while.*

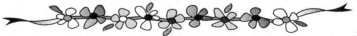

The health of the people is really the foundation upon which all their happiness and all their powers as a state depend. – Benjamin Disraeli

Nothing transforms anyone as much as changing from a negative to a positive attitude and positive actions.

It's a shame millions suffer from ignorance!

IT'S IMPORTANT TO EXERCISE THE STOMACH MUSCLES

Most people have allowed their stomach muscles to become flabby. A good time to start strengthening these abdominal muscles (your natural girdle of muscles) and getting them under control is first thing in the morning, when you are in bed.

Lying on your back . . . with nothing over you but a thin sheet . . . fix your eyes and attention upon your abdomen. Now start a movement of its muscles . . . any kind of movement possible at first. Try to bring the contents of the abdomen upwards, then force them downwards. Wiggle your insides, toss them in one direction, then another, then from side to side. When you discover you can control them in one direction, practice that set of muscles, then try to get the muscles to twist and turn another way. Thinking about and using these muscles is the beginning.

The point you need to reach is that of controlling the abdominal muscles in the same way you do those of the legs and arms. Your stomach muscles must do your bidding, if you want to develop a useful diaphragm. After you have obtained some control over your stomach muscles while lying on your back in bed, *begin doing the same movements while standing upright.* You can accomplish much more in this upright position.

Upright, with hands passively hanging at your sides, draw up the contents of the abdomen until it looks like a deep valley, as though everything inside of you were up in the chest cavity. Then push them down until you are laughingly and innocently ashamed of your protruding belly. Draw up, push down, suck in, wiggle, twist and then tighten your midsection.

When you acquire this willpower over the abdominal muscles and contents, you will discover that you will also establish a more normal bowel rhythm. Usually upon arising and an hour after each meal, there will be a bowel movement. See pages 45 and 56 to improve your elimination.

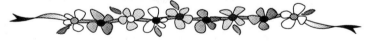

Your waistline is your healthline, dateline and ageline. – Patricia Bragg

---

God gave His creatures light and air and water open to the skies;
Man locks himself in a stifling lair and wonders why his brother dies.
– Oliver Wendall Holmes

DIAPHRAGM EXERCISE

In exercising your abdominal muscles, you will also be exercising your diaphragm . . . especially in the upward and downward pushing movements. You should do this special exercise for your diaphragm. *Locate your diaphragm* by placing one hand at your waistline, then, holding the other palm upward in front of your mouth, blow imaginary dust from the palm. Where you feel a strong muscular contraction when blowing, that's your **diaphragm, the most important muscle in correct Bragg Super Power Breathing.**

Now walk around your room on your tiptoes . . . with your hands reaching high over your head. Raise your diaphragm as high as your strength will allow you to lift it. Press it against your lungs and force out every bit of carbon dioxide-laden air. This is a super lung cleanser. **Try it now.**

Then push your diaphragm down and out against the walls of your waistline. Feel it stretch the muscles of your chest and abdomen and suck the oxygen-bearing fresh air deeply and slowly into your lungs with your chest lifted high.

If you feel a little dizzy at the oxygen stimulation, stop for a moment, then continue. *Begin by doing this exercise five times . . . gradually increasing to ten.* When you are able to do this exercise with ease and pleasure, you are ready to start your Bragg Super Power Breathing Program.

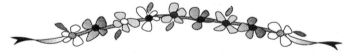

Be healthy and happy. Stretch yourselves for more body freedom, for greatness and for height. – Patricia Bragg

---

Who you are speaks so loudly, I can't hear what you're saying. – Ralph Waldo Emerson

---

I've studied, researched, listened, pondered and questioned what worked, why and how. – Amy Graham

---

Learning is finding out what you already know. Doing is demonstrating that you know it. Teaching is reminding others that they know it just as well as you. You are all learners, doers, teachers. – Richard Bach

---

The sense of obligation to continue is present in all of us. A duty to strive is the duty of us all. I felt a call to that duty. – Abraham Lincoln

Chapter 7

What Is Bragg Super Power Breathing?

Bragg Super Power Breathing is based upon simple, natural laws. The more oxygen you get into the body, the more carbon dioxide poison you will eliminate from the body. When oxygen replaces carbon dioxide, there will be greater purity of the blood, cells and organs of the body for health.

It is a well known scientific fact that when all known modern methods of healing fail, that oxygen is used. Thousands upon thousands of lives have been saved with oxygen.

Then let's reason this way: If a preponderance of oxygen can save the lives of humans who are on the brink of death, is it not logical that more oxygen can prolong our lives . . . that it will free us from poisons that bring pain and distress to our physical bodies . . . and, above all, give us a greater enjoyment in living?

Oxygen is the only stimulant upon which you can safely rely as a depression chaser and body builder. **Bragg Super Power Breathing has one purpose . . . and that is the forcing of more life-giving oxygen into all parts of the body.**

Bragg Super Power Breathing Exercises should not be confused with physical exercises. While this Breathing does produce more energy and physical and nerve strength, it has nothing to do with mere muscular development. However, it is almost impossible to have ample oxygen freely circulating in the body without its beneficial effects occurring throughout the body. Extra benefits will be healthier muscle-tone and more firmness of the flesh. Oxygen is a wonderful normalizer.

The basic principle of Bragg Super Power Breathing is to fill the lungs to capacity with oxygen and hold in the breath while leaning forward and dropping the head below the heart. This forces the oxygenated blood by force of gravity into the cavities of the head to energize your brain center.

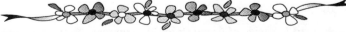

Bragg Super Power Breathing of longer, slower, deep breaths will help produce a more vital, youthful, longer life for you! – Paul C. Bragg

BRAGG EXERCISES STIMULATE THE PITUITARY GLAND

Stimulation of the body's master gland, the pituitary, is the first and greatest benefit of Super Power Breathing Exercises. Located at the base of the brain, the pituitary gland is the master of every human act and unconscious function occurring within the heart and abdominal cavity. It also determines a person's height, length of bones, muscle strength, mental sharpness, pulse strength and lifespan.

The pituitary is *the master gland of life and* controls the functions of all the other body glands. **The more oxygenated blood you give the pituitary gland, the greater the output of all the valuable hormones of the body.** The better the glands function, the more the body will rejuvenate itself.

That is why these seven exercises which I am giving you are called Super Power Breathing Exercises. Although each is directed toward a specific part of the body, all employ the same basic, super oxygen principle . . . and all stimulate the master pituitary gland and brain area.

EARLY MORNING IS THE BEST TIME TO BEGIN SUPER POWER BREATHING EXERCISES

I recommend a ten to fifteen minute period early in the morning for your Super Power Breathing Exercises. After you have awakened your body with a few preliminary stretching exercises, sip a glass of distilled water or our delicious Bragg Apple Cider Vinegar Cocktail ✳*(1 – 2 tsp ACV and 1– 2 tsp raw honey in glass of distilled water)*, then get ready to start your day with a peak supply of energy by doing Super Power Breathing.

The early morning hours are especially important for these exercises if you are a city-dweller because the air is less polluted at this time of day than any other. Start your day with a glowing sense of well-being and a store of energy to carry you through whatever work you have to do and problems you may meet. Your energy level will zoom up!

Think of this health-building period with pleasant anticipation. It's a time to build your vitality, energy, strength and all the good things that come to a healthy body. Your faithful efforts will return super results. Go into it with dedicated self-responsibility and enthusiasm.

✳ Read *Miracles of Apple Cider Vinegar* and *The Water Book*.
(See back pages for Bragg Book info)

40

FRESH AIR AND WARMTH NECESSARY

Sleep in a well ventilated (airy) room on a firm mattress with cotton percale or cotton flannel sheets, and the same natural fabrics for nightwear is preferable. Do not use heating blankets or heating pads, as these disturb your body's natural currents and can even be harmful to your health, according to scientists. A hot water bottle is safer.

Be sure there's ample fresh air in your room or you can do these exercises before an open window. I want you to get full benefit of this wonderful stimulation and to enjoy every minute of it. If it's too cool when you get out of bed, put on something that is loose and warm. I often wear a sweat shirt and pants.

As you start doing your exercises you will soon feel a wonderful circulation glow coming over your entire body . . . and you will become warm. As soon as you feel warm enough, peel off your sweat clothes and get right down to your bare skin. Give yourself an outside as well as an inside air bath. Let the 96 million pores of your skin breathe in the breath of life also. Remember, you also breathe through your skin! It's an important organ of respiration – often called your *third lung.*

The pores of your body will welcome a plunge into real fresh air. They are going to be wrapped up in clothes all day and probably at night, too, unless you sleep nude. A daily air bath does wonders for your skin; no creams or lotions can give you . . . *skin you love to touch . . .* like fresh air can.

A daily private air bath also greatly enhances your skin's primary function as the thermostatic control of your body temperature. You will help condition it to meet hot and cold weather perfectly. It's a faithful thermostat when you treat it well. But if you keep your body over-clothed and overheated all the time, your skin becomes like a hot-house plant, unable to withstand drastic temperature changes. When you allow your entire body to breathe freely in the buff, your body thermostat learns to adjust and will work for you in both hot and cold weather.

He who cannot find time for exercise will have to find time for illness.
– Lord Derby

Rare Centenarian Couple: *I wish everyone would realize it's never too late to turn your life around for the better and maintain a love life!*
– Jay and Lila Hoover, 100 and 101 years young of Parma, Idaho

41

BREATHE THROUGH THE MOUTH AND NOSE

Let me make it clear that in normal breathing, one should breathe through the mouth and nose. Nature has equipped your nose with hair filters to strain out dust and soot, temperature regulating chambers (sinuses) to warm or cool the air before it enters the lungs, and moist mucous to trap particles which pass through the hair filters to be expelled through the nose or mouth.

But Nature has also equipped the human body with a larger, secondary air entrance (the mouth) for use when a greater amount of oxygen is needed . . . as in strenuous exercise such as swimming, running, bicycling, tennis. etc.

Since the purpose of Super Power Breathing is to take into the lungs as much oxygen as possible, we use both the nose and mouth to breathe in and out. *Pucker the lips into a small opening, and inhale slowly and strongly with a hissing sound.*

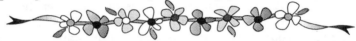

You can always remember that you have the following good reasons for living the Bragg Healthy Lifestyle:

- The ironclad laws of Mother Nature and God.
- Your common sense which tells you that you are doing right.
- Your aim to make your health better, stronger and your life longer.
- Your resolve to prevent illness so that you may enjoy life to the fullest.
- By making an art of healthy living, you will be youthful at any age.
- You will retain your faculties and be hale, hearty, active and useful far beyond the ordinary length of years, and you will also possess superior mental, emotional and physical powers.

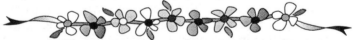

WANTED – For Robbing Health & Life	
KILLER Saturated Fats	CHOKER Hydrogenated Fats
CLOGGER Salt	DEADEYED Devitalized Foods
DOPEY Caffeine	HARD (Inorganic Minerals) Water
PLUGGER Frying Pan	CRAZY Alcohol
DEATH-DEALER Drugs	SMOKEY Tobacco
JERKEY Turbulent Emotions	LOAFER Laziness
GREASY Overweight	HOGGY Over-Eating

Chapter 8

Bragg Super Power Breathing Exercises

EXERCISE NO. 1 – CLEANSING BREATH

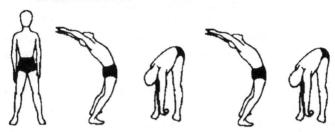

This is your basic Super Power Breathing Exercise.

Stand erect, feet about 15 to 18 inches apart, hands and arms relaxed at your sides.

Raise the hands overhead. Now bend forward as far as possible . . . keeping the knees slightly bent and relaxed . . . at the same time exhaling through the mouth. Compress your chest and push upward with your diaphragm and abdominal muscles to expel every bit of carbon dioxide from your lungs.

Now slowly inhale through your nose and mouth, pushing downward with your diaphragm and expanding your chest at front and sides to draw in the air to the full capacity of your lungs as you return to the standing position, bringing your arms upward in a half-circle to the overhead position.

NOTE: All Super Power Breathing Exercises begin this way.

To complete the Cleansing Breath Exercise: As your hands reach the overhead position, tighten your diaphragm and hold your breath for four or five seconds (mentally counting, *One thousand one, one thousand two*, etc.) while pulling your abdominal muscles back as if to pin your stomach to your backbone. Then exhale completely while bending forward as at the beginning, and inhale as you return to the starting position. Do this exercise five times.

Exercise with a receptive body, not a striving mind. – Yoga Texts

EXERCISE No. 2 – THE SUPER BRAIN-POWER BREATH

Start by exhaling and inhaling in Exercise No. 1. When your hands reach the overhead position, hold your breath (hold nose closed if necessary) and bend forward from the waist, knees bent, dropping your head downward as far as possible. Continue to hold your breath to the count of ten (mentally counting, *One thousand one, one thousand two . . .* etc.). The purpose of this exercise is to allow the oxygen-filled blood to suffuse the pituitary gland and reach, refresh and recharge every part of your brain for sharper thinking, as well as cleanse the skull cavities (sinuses, ears, nose, eyes, mouth).

Holding your breath, return to standing position, then bend forward, exhaling vigorously through the mouth. Slowly inhale as you return to starting position. Do this exercise five times at the beginning, gradually increase to ten times.

NOTE: As previously mentioned, you may not be able to hold your breath for the full count at first. If you feel dizzy, exhale, return to standing position, drop arms to sides and relax for a minute or two before continuing the exercise. You will gradually build your oxygen tolerance to the full count.

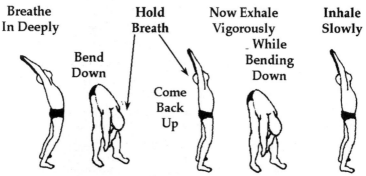

EXERCISE No. 3 – SUPER-KIDNEY BREATH

Locate your kidneys on the lower back, just below the end of your rib cage near the waistline. Get the *feel* of them by placing your palms over this area, fingers and thumbs pointed downward . . . as this is the position you will take during the breath-holding part of this exercise.

Exhale and inhale as at the beginning of Exercise No. 1. As your hands reach the overhead position, tighten your diaphragm and pin your stomach to your backbone with your abdominal muscles, while holding your breath, and then firmly place palms, with light pressure, over kidneys (on back below waist) and bend backward for a silent count of 10 (*One thousand one . . .* etc.).

Still holding your breath, return to standing position, bend forward, exhaling vigorously through the mouth. Slowly inhale as you return to the starting position. Do this exercise five times at the start, gradually increasing to ten. (Use the same precaution in breath-holding count as previously given.)

EXERCISE No. 4 - BLOWING THE BOWEL

This exercise should be done in the bathroom soon after rising each morning, and several times within an hour after eating. If you will make this a habit, you will soon find that you will get a bowel movement within an hour after eating. This is as it usually should be: outgo equals intake.

Exhale and inhale as at the beginning of Exercise No. 1. Now, holding your breath, drop hands to sides in a relaxed position and slowly go into a squatting position, then strain for a bowel movement for the silent count of several seconds. Return to standing position and complete exercise by exhaling and inhaling as in previous exercises.

Squatting is the natural way to have a bowel movement. It opens up the anal area more directly. When on the toilet putting your feet up on a waste basket or footstool will give you the same effect.

EXERCISE No. 5 - FILLING THE LUNGS

This exercise is to get oxygen into the little-used air sacs at the bottom (apex) of the lungs, down near your waistline.

Exhale and inhale as at the start of Exercise No. 1, but instead of returning arms to overhead position, drop them relaxed at sides, bring feet together, toes and heels touching.

Holding your breath, bend to the right and reach towards the floor with the fingers of your right hand, at the same time bringing the left hand up to touch under the left armpit. Hold position for a silent count of ten.

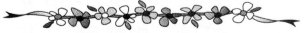

The unexamined life is not worth living. It is a time to reevaluate your past as a guide to your new, fresh future. – Socrates

45

Return to starting position, exhale and inhale as before, then repeat breath-holding position on the left side, reaching toward the floor with the left hand, and touching the right hand under the right armpit for a count of ten. Do this exercise five to ten times, alternating from side to side.

EXERCISE No. 6 – THE LIVER CLEANSE BREATH

Exhale and inhale as at the beginning of Exercise No. 1. Now bring the feet together and clasp the fingers overhead, palms upward. Keep legs stiff from the hips down and, holding the breath, bend slowly to the right side with as much stretch as possible, then bend slowly to the left with a good stretch, alternating these bends to right and left five times, each time holding your breath.

Return to starting position with feet apart. Exhale and inhale with the usual forward bend. Do this five times – gradually increasing to ten times.

EXERCISE No. 7 – HEART STRENGTHENER

The purpose of this exercise is to expand the aorta, the main trunk of the arterial system which carries blood from the heart after it has been oxygenated by Super Power Breathing. This exercise stimulates the circulation of blood in the heart, as well as throughout the rest of the body, helping to increase the power of the entire cardiovascular respiratory function. This exercise may give relief to those who suffer from the feelings of suffocation and apprehension caused by angina pectoris. See page 56 for Healthy Heart Advice.

This exercise starts with the same exhaling and inhaling as in the beginning of Exercise No. 1, except that the arms are held forward at shoulder height (not overhead). When you return to the standing position, hold your breath – clasp your nose tightly with thumb and index finger so that no air escapes – pretend you are blowing your nose. You should feel some air pressure in your ears.

Now, with knees bent, bend over from the waist, and gently bring your head down below your heart and waist, and continue to hold your breath for a silent count of ten.

Return to the starting position and exhale and inhale in the usual Super Power Breathing manner. Repeat this exercise five times, gradually increasing to ten times.

FAITHFULNESS COUNTS TOWARDS SUPER HEALTH

Every person who is interested in Super Health should take time each morning to do these Super Power Breathing Exercises. Take your present physical condition into consideration when you start on this program. Go slowly at first. A large part of your lungs has probably been dormant for some time. It will take time to open up these areas.

Make these exercises a daily habit. Make them as much a part of your life as dressing and brushing your teeth. The wonderful results you will obtain from faithfully following these exercises will repay you many times over in more abundant super health and energy, peace and longevity!

WE THANK THEE

For flowers that bloom about our feet;
For song of bird and hum of bee;
For all things fair we hear or see,
Father in heaven we thank Thee!
For blue of stream and blue of sky;
For pleasant shade of branches high;
For fragrant air and cooling breeze;
For beauty of the blooming trees
Father in heaven we thank Thee!
For mother love and father care,
For brothers strong and sisters fair;
For love at home and here each day;
For guidance lest we go astray,
Father in heaven we thank Thee!
For this new morning with its light;
For rest and shelter of the night;
For health and food, for love and friends;
For every thing His goodness sends
Father in heaven we thank Thee!
— Ralph Waldo Emerson

Take time for 12 things

1 Take time to **Work** –
   it is the price of success.

2 Take time to **Think** –
   it is the source of power.

3 Take time to **Play** –
   it is the secret of youth.

4 Take time to **Read** –
   it is the foundation of knowledge.

5 Take time to **Worship** –
   it is the highway of reverence and
   washes the dust of earth from our eyes.

6 Take time to **Help and Enjoy Friends** –
   it is the source of happiness.

7 Take time to **Love** –
   it is the one sacrament of life.

8 Take time to **Dream** –
   it hitches the soul to the stars.

9 Take time to **Laugh** –
   it is the singing that helps life's loads.

10 Take time for **Beauty** –
   it is everywhere in nature.

11 Take time for **Health** –
   it is the true wealth and treasure of life.

12 Take time to **Plan** –
   it is the secret of being able to have time
   to take time for the first eleven things.

Teach me Thy way O Lord, and Lead me in Thy plain path.
– Psalms 27:11

Chapter 9

Learn To Control Your Breathing

Your lungs will hold at least six pints of air. If you keep your lungs filled to capacity you will feel better, have more energy, suffer less fatigue, sleep better, wake up faster, and be a happier person. With practice you can learn to control your breathing, so that you will take only six to eight long, full breaths per minute and add more healthy years to your life!

EVENING AND BEDTIME ROUTINES

At the end of the day's heavier activities, make it a habit to refresh yourself with some stretching, diaphragm exercises and a few Super Power Breaths. This helps cleanse the dust and impurities from your body which have accumulated throughout the day. Make as much space as possible for oxygen, then you will have a relaxed and healthier evening.

Just before going to bed, after you have removed your clothing, stretch every inch of your body and exhale with vigor and slowly and deeply inhale with ease. Then get into bed and let the food of your evening meal be ground up, separated and its valuable life-giving nutrients go to their proper places.

BREATHING TO RELIEVE PAIN

Civilized human beings with unhealthy eating and living habits tend to accumulate latent poisons in their bodies. That means that Nature has concentrated toxic poisons in different parts of the body at periods during life when these could not be disposed of through the regular avenues of elimination. These poisons are stored in veins, arteries, joints and organs. When they press on the nerves, there is pain. You may think this is something new . . . but, except in cases of direct injury, it is usually a *flare up* of old stored-up toxic poisons.

Don't take pills to ease warning pains, eliminate the cause! Live The Bragg Healthy Lifestyle! Let oxygen help burn the poisons out of your body! There is absolutely no better way of flushing poisons out of the body than by the powerful action of oxygen. Ample oxygen and drinking eight glasses of pure distilled water daily are the greatest purifiers on earth!

For instance, you may have a pain in your right foot. That is quite common, since by force of gravity poisons will many times seek the lowest level of the body. Example: gout.

Now let's get the toxic poison out of that right foot. The technique is as follows: Lie flat on the floor, take a long, deep breath and hold it. While you are holding your breath, raise the left leg, bent at the knee, and with both hands pull and press your leg against your chest at the same time using the downward force of your diaphragm. You will feel the oxygenated blood flowing down into your unrestricted right foot.

This same technique may be applied to any part of the body. For example, for a headache, take the full breath (exhaling and inhaling as at the start of Exercise No. 1) Holding the breath, bend downward as far as you can. This allows a free flow of oxygenated blood to the cavities of the head and brain.

Aches and pains from fatigue are nearly always due to stagnant venous blood that is filled with carbon dioxide and congested at various parts of the body. Swollen ankles, for instance, are generally due to an accumulation of venous blood. Exercise and super power breathing help to activate the circulation and return this blood to the heart to be pumped to the lungs, where the carbon dioxide will be exchanged for purifying oxygen. If you have been sitting or standing for a long time and your ankles become swollen, lie flat on your back on the floor, raise your legs and stretch your feet toward the ceiling and breathe deeply. You will feel the blood flowing from your feet and ankles toward your heart. If you are in a place where you cannot do this, breathe deeply and hold your breath while you alternately rise up on your toes, then down and up on your heels. The deep breathing and muscular action will stimulate circulation and relieve the venous blood congestion and take the ache out of your feet!

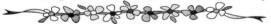

You can increase the oxygen currents of nerve force with the breath, and send it to heal parts of your body. – Paul C. Bragg

RHYTHMIC BRAGG SUPER POWER BREATHING AND BRISK WALKING ARE POWERFUL HEALTH BUILDERS

Of all forms of exercise, brisk walking is the one that brings most of the body into action. It is the *king of exercise* and when the rhythm of your deep breathing and the rhythm of your stride are in harmony, you feel like a winner!

Practice these Breathing Exercises faithfully to gain perfect control of your breathing and become a tireless walker. As the oxygen-filled blood courses through your body, your legs will carry you along buoyantly. Walk tall with head high, back straight, chest up, tummy in, arms swinging easily from your shoulders, legs moving smoothly as though they were attached to the middle of your torso.

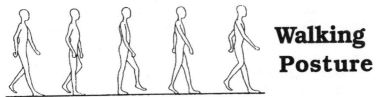

Walking Posture

Always prepare a new foot base before leaving the old.

Enjoy your walk. Set your own pace, with a free spirit and a light heart. Watch with interest the things and people you pass . . . or let your walking be an accompaniment to your ideas and thoughts. As you breathe and walk rhythmically you lose awareness of your body, and you become as near poet and philosopher as you will ever be.

You can truly *walk your worries away!* As the blood courses through your arteries and veins cleansing and nourishing your entire body, you become filled with a sense of well-being that cleanses your mind of its troubles and nourishes it with positive, healthy, happy thoughts.

As I stride along on my walks I say, *Health, Strength, Youth, Vitality, Peace, Love and Joy!*

You should walk briskly at least one to two miles every day and more when you have time! Don't give yourself excuses! Make your daily walk a fixed item in any kind of weather. In stormy weather walk in your home, on your porch or driveway, in the mall, etc. When traveling use hotel hallways, stairs or even the treadmill or health rider in the hotel's gym. Walking can be done anytime during your waking hours. Start today!

Dad and I always preferred outdoor walking, but walking indoors is far better than none at all. When traveling around the world on my lecture tours, I often take a light jog or a brisk evening walk through the corridors and up and down the stairs of my hotel. My favorite places to walk briskly are beaches, hills and the open decks of ocean cruise ships.

> Brisk walking is the king of exercise. With walking you discover the beauty of nature and it awakens, softens and enriches your soul and life! – Patricia Bragg

WALKING BUILDS NEW BLOOD VESSELS

The June 1995 edition of *American Health* reported that Dr. Gary Giangola, a vascular surgeon at New York University Medical Center, prescribed walking instead of bypass surgery for a patient's atherosclerosis that was so pervasive it had severely restricted the blood flow to his legs and was causing extreme pain and numbness in his feet. Dr. Giangola told his patient that if he walked one mile every day (even if that meant stopping every two blocks to recover), he would build new blood vessels (collaterals) which would bypass his closed arteries. One year later the patient was able to walk several miles easily . Walking and a healthy lifestyle usually provide a permanent cure! The results of surgery are often risky, life-threatening and temporary at best, unless it is combined with lifestyle changes, including a healthy diet and exercise!

SUPER POWER BREATHING MAKES EXERCISE JOYOUS

Whether your preferred exercise is walking, hiking, jogging, biking, aerobics, swimming, golfing, dancing, calisthenics, tennis, weightlifting, or any other aerobic activity, you will reap greater benefits from it. when you establish the correct habits of Bragg Super Power Breathing. What's more, you'll have more energy to exercise and you will enjoy it more!

> The Bragg Bible of Health and Fitness, *The Complete Fitness Manual,* will give you the Bragg complete program. It's 600 pages for super fitness. Also read these other Bragg Healthy Lifestyle Books: *Keep The Heart Healthy and Fit, The Miracle of Fasting, The Fitness/Spine Motion* and *The Miracles of Apple Cider Vinegar.* (See back pages for Bragg Book info.)

DEEP BREATHING HAS CALMING EFFECT ON THE NERVES

The greatest tranquilizer for jangled nerves is deep, slow, diaphragmatic breathing. Today's tensions and pressures put additional strain on our nervous systems, and the condition is aggravated by poor posture habits and shallow breathing. Your Bragg Super Power Breathing Program will help you correct both of these unhealthy habits . . . and have a calming, healthy effect on your nervous system and entire body!

During your workday, take at least a minute out of every hour to pause and s-t-r-e-t-c-h from your toes to the top of your head while doing deep, diaphragmatic breathing. Do back and forward shoulder rolls. The small amount of time invested in this will save you a great deal of time during the day, because you will be able to do your work faster and with greater efficiency. This is particularly important for a desk worker, but it is also helpful in any kind of work, even manual labor.

By oxygenating and relaxing your nerves, you will find that petty annoyances on the job and irritations with fellow workers or the boss will not ruffle and upset you!

Whenever a big emotional upset occurs – as it inevitably does at times with all of us . . . go off by yourself and take long, full diaphragmatic breaths. See how few long, slow breaths you can take in a minute. You will find your nerves quieting down and logical thinking will replace emotionalism. You will become master of the situation, and you will be able to resolve your problem more calmly.

To help relieve stress, please read our Bragg Book, *Building Powerful Nerve Force.* (See back pages for Bragg Book information.

RELIEF IN RESPIRATORY AILMENTS WITH DEEP BREATHING

Letters and case histories in our files give testimony to the blessed relief that Bragg Super Power Breathing has brought to literally thousands of sufferers with breathing problems such as sinusitis, bronchitis, asthma and emphysema.

These suffocating diseases, characterized by inflammation of the mucous membranes and obstruction of the air passages, have become more and more prevalent today as our air becomes more polluted. In fact, sinusitis, inflammation of the mucous membrane lining of the sinus cavities in the head, is one of the most common illnesses seen by doctors today.

Many people suffering from these respiratory complaints fail to understand that these are naturally occurring body responses to an unhealthy environment. They are hoping nasal sprays will relieve their symptoms. Many don't follow directions and abuse the sprays, often becoming addicted to the spray with disastrous consequences. Nasal spray abuse can cause a secondary illness: *rhinitis medicamentosa,* in which the patient's nose is inflamed by the medicine itself.

To help relieve these symptoms naturally try an Apple Cider Vinegar nasal sniff wash. (1 tsp ACV per cup of warm distilled water. Put it in your hand, inhale gently up nostrils.) Also drink your ACV Health Cocktail (recipe on page 63) three times a day. Use air purifiers or humidifiers and don't lie flat on your back.

When people contract bronchitis and asthma, the mucous membranes of their bronchial tubes become inflamed. The human computer triggers the release of more mucus in an attempt to soothe and heal the irritation, but unless this mucus is decongested and expelled, it clogs these vital air passages. In asthma, even the tiny bronchioles (the smallest branches of bronchial tubes in the air sacs) become swollen. Victims feel as though they are suffocating, and in severe cases, they do!

Prolonged chronic bronchitis or asthma can progress into emphysema, in which the air sacs become so distended with trapped air that this delicate tissue loses its vital elasticity. The air sacs themselves suffocate, one by one.

Super Power Breathing cannot restore tissue that has been destroyed, but it can help salvage and revitalize the rest of the lungs! The life-giving inflow of oxygen acts as a natural decongestant – gradually clearing the bronchioles and bronchial tubes, removing carbon dioxide and other wastes from the air sacs and all the lung tissues, and helping revitalize every possible cell with oxygen and nutrients.

Along with the Super Power Breathing, it is absolutely essential that you eliminate all milk and milk products from your diet, as these are mucus-forming. This includes yogurt, cheeses of all kinds, butter, ice cream, milk puddings, etc.

Each birthday is the beginning of your own personal New Year.
Your chance to begin anew, to take a fresh, new healthy grip on life.
– Paul C. Bragg

Many victims of these respiratory ailments have gained permanent relief by following The Bragg Healthy Lifestyle. Faithfully follow the Bragg Super Power Breathing Program and gradually increase the amount of brisk walking and other exercise, fast for a 24 hour period every week, and eat a diet consisting of healthy, live foods. Also read page 98 for important supplements to take. We suggest you read these Bragg Books: *Miracle of Fasting, The Toxicless Diet Purification and Healing System* and *The Miracles of Apple Cider Vinegar*.

HELP FOR ASTHMA ATTACKS

Contrary to common belief, asthma attacks are not caused by an inability to breathe (inhale), but rather by an inability to exhale the dirty air collected in the lungs. Try the following technique for relief of an asthma attack. Someone else needs to learn this technique, because you cannot do it for yourself.

Stand behind the person having the attack, wrap your arms around the torso in a hug, then using both hands, lift the entire tummy and diaphragm upward, as if you were trying to push it up under the ribs and breastbone. (This is much like the Heimlich maneuver for a choking person.) When the person can breathe again, have her get down on her hands and knees, straddle her and repeat the process. This position helps the diaphragm return to its normal, healthy position easily. Naturally, if the attack is severe and this technique does not work, be sure to follow your regular medical program.

CONTROLLED BREATHING EXERCISE
FOR SUPER OXYGEN AND SUPER HEALTH

Do this exercise before getting out of bed in the morning and throughout your day, whenever you can take a minute or two. Count to yourself as you gently exhale and then slowly inhale. As you become more practiced you will increase the count. It's challenging to have breathing contests with friends and family to see who can take the deepest, slowest, longest breaths. This exercise will strengthen your lungs, chest and all the muscles around your midwaist and will improve your lung capacity and super breathing power. It will give you a firmer, trimmer waistline. This will help you learn to breathe with control in and out (vary breathing through mouth and nose.). When on walks pay attention to how long it takes to inhale – ideally your exhale should be longer.

DIAPHRAGMATIC BREATHING SUPER OXYGENATOR

Raise your arms so that your ribs are separated. Rather than breathe as you normally would, pant while breathing. Pant until your diaphragm is tired. Your exhale panting should take about twice as long as your inhale. For example, if your inhale lasts for a count of six, try to make your exhale last to twelve. Do this exercise daily especially before retiring. This will help re-oxygenate your entire body and help remove toxins from your system so you can enjoy more super health.

CORRECT BREATHING BENEFITS CHILDBIRTH, MOTHER & BABY

In natural childbirth classes parents are taught certain breathing techniques, such as the Lamaze or Bradley methods, which make childbirth less uncomfortable. Mothers who have practice Bragg Super Power Breathing throughout their pregnancies have stronger muscles, greatly enhancing their ability to use these specific techniques and generally making the birth process easier. This ensures that the mother and the baby will have a happier, healthier birth experience.

The primary benefits for the mother are a shortened recovery time and the ability to fully participate in the joyful process of her child's birth. For the baby the primary benefit comes from the well-oxygenated blood the mother has been providing for the nine months she carried the baby in her womb. **This oxygen helps prevent birth defects and helps ensure that the baby is born healthy and ready for life!**

ONE-BREATH MEDITATION WORKS MIRACLES

ATP (adenosine triphosphate) is a naturally occurring by-product of breathing that regulates action, thought and feeling. A dip in ATP levels can cause fatigue, aches and pains. One breath meditation reverses falling levels of ATP.

1. Sit in a comfortable chair and straighten your back, shoulders back and relaxed.
2. Inhale slowly and deeply, clear your mind completely. Relax your shoulders and imagine yourself deeply drawing vitality from the oxygen rich air.
3. Hold the breath for a moment, then exhale slowly and deeply, releasing every bit of tension from your muscles.

Use this one minute refresher throughout the day as needed to restore your body, mind and soul.

Chapter 10

The Problem of Air Pollution

Practically every city today faces the problem of polluted air. If you are a city dweller . . . as most people are . . . how are you to get the full, healthy benefit of oxygen?

Do your Super Power Breathing Exercises early in the morning when the air is cleaner and less contaminated.

If you live in a smoggy area, it's important to install the best air filters you can find. We did this for our Hollywood home. Learn how to clean the filters and replace the pads, so they are always clean, washed, and able to do their job of cleaning and washing the air. Buy filter pads in long strips and cut them to fit as needed.

We finally sold our Hollywood home because we did not want to live in smog or any kind of polluted air even for short periods of time. If you are able to move away from pollution, do so! Your entire being benefits from fresh, clean air!

CONSERVE OXYGEN WITH VITAMIN E

You should also fortify yourself internally with Vitamin E (natural d-alpha tocopherol), the body's *oxygen monitor*. One of the vital functions of this *wonder vitamin* is to regulate the use of oxygen by the body cells – assuring that every bit of life-giving oxygen is properly utilized for essential energy, with a reserve retained in the red corpuscles for use when extra effort is needed. In this way Vitamin E increases the energy potential of every bit of oxygen you breathe by 25 to 50 percent, according to documented medical research.

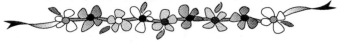

Man is composed of such elements as vital breath, deeds, thoughts and the senses. – The Upanishads

My father and I have certainly found this true in athletes who have trained under our instruction. Murray Rose, for example, the youngest Olympic triple gold medal winner in history, who eventually won six Olympic medals in distance swimming, took a minimum of 200 I.U.'s of Vitamin E daily and increased his intake to 1500 I.U.'s during competition. In fact, wheatgerm, a prime power source of Vitamin E, is an integral part of the training of outstanding athletes.

Many decades ago when my health pioneer father first introduced to America the important need for wheatgerm and Vitamin E supplements, he was called a *faddist* and a *health nut*. It's gratifying that finally today, in these turbulent health care times, his health teachings have been substantiated by thorough scientific research, both laboratory and clinical, in the fields of biochemistry, exercise, nutrition and medicine.

It is tragic, however, that it took over seventy years and thousands of needless premature deaths and the overall deterioration of health throughout America and the civilized world before people realized that they rob themselves of the *staff of life* when they make bread from refined white flour. White flour has been stripped of its precious wheatgerm, one of the primary sources of Vitamin E in the human diet. It can be categorically stated that everyone who subsists on the standard *civilized* diet, devoid of whole grains but replete with refined white flour products, is suffering from Vitamin E deficiency. This means everyone of any age from infancy through childhood and adolescence to adulthood.

Widespread Vitamin E deficiency has been documented as the prime factor in the disastrous increase in heart attacks and other cardiovascular problems. Brothers, Dr. Evan Shute and Dr. Wilfrid Shute, at the Shute Institute in London, Ontario, Canada, conducted thorough clinical research for over 30 years, treating over 30,000 cardiovascular patients with massive doses of Vitamin E (alpha tocopherol) from natural sources with amazing success. Their extensive work has been confirmed, contributed to and extended by hundreds of physicians and biochemists throughout the world.

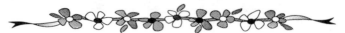

God sends the food; man by refining and processing foods destroys its nutritional value. Eat only God's healthy, natural foods. – Patricia Bragg

The primary functions of Vitamin E in the human body have been established as those regulating and maintaining the health of the entire cardiovascular system. Vitamin E plays a vital role in the body's defense against air pollution. It conserves oxygen within the body cells and bloodstream

The possibility of using Vitamin E as an *antidote to smog* has been researched by Dr. Aloys L. Tappel, Professor of Biochemistry at the University of California, Davis. He also believes that this natural anti-oxidation property of Vitamin E can help reverse the ageing process and recommends Vitamin E supplements to help promote a healthier and longer life for everyone. Read page 98 for more info on supplements.

This oxygen conservation quality of Vitamin E may also be effective in the relief or control of emphysema, the deadly disease of lung deterioration which has become increasingly more prevalent as our air has become more contaminated.

Vitamin E is an amazingly effective treatment for burns of all degrees, and a Vitamin E salve is now available for home application to minor burns, sunburn and skin problems.

ADD WONDER-WORKING VITAMIN E TO YOUR DIET

Natural Vitamin E Supplements are available at Health Stores. If you are just starting on Vitamin E, doctors recommend that you begin with 100 I.U.'s daily, gradually increasing to 400 for women and 600 for men.

Raw wheatgerm is an excellent natural source of Vitamin E. Raw wheatgerm and wheatgerm oil are available at Health Stores. Both must be refrigerated immediately after opening! Wheatgerm is highly perishable – that's why commercial millers refine it out of your flour. Apparently, they're more interested in the shelf life of their product than in the length and quality of your life.

In the Bragg household, we sprinkle raw wheatgerm over stewed or fresh fruit and often over fresh raw vegetable salads. It has a pleasant, nutty taste. If you like the taste of wheatgerm oil (some do, some don't), you will enjoy using it in your salad dressing. Mothers can even add wheatgerm oil to the baby's milk. Clint Eastwood's two healthy children both thrived on wheatgerm oil added to their goat's milk (1/4 tsp per cup), after they were weaned at one year.

FOODS RICH IN WONDERWORKING VITAMIN E

A nutritious variety of foods contain notable amounts of oxygen-saving Vitamin E. The following table was compiled from lists in the authoritative *Bridges Food & Beverage Analyses*.

FOOD	QUANTITY	VIT. E I.Us.
Apples	1 medium	.74
Bananas	1 medium	.40
Barley	1/2 cup	4.20
Beans, Dry Navy	1/2 cup steamed	3.60
Beef Steak	1 average piece	.63
Beef Liver	1 average piece	1.40
Butter	6 tablespoons	2.40
Carrots	1 cup	.45
Celery, Green	1/2 cup	2.60
Chicken	3 slices	.25
Corn, Dried	1 cup	20.00
Cornmeal, Yellow	1/2 cup	1.70
Corn Oil	6 tablespoons	87.00
Eggs, Whole Fertile	2	2.00
Endive, Escarole	1/2 cup	2.00
Flour, Whole Grain	1 cup	54.00
Grapefruit	1/2	.52
Haddock	1 average piece	.39
Kale	1/2 cup	8.00
Lamb Chops	2 rib chops	.77
Lettuce	6 leaves	.50
Mackerel, canned	1/2 cup	205.00
Oatmeal, cooked	1/2 cup	2.00
Olive Oil	1/2 cup	5.00
Onions, raw	2 medium	.26
Oranges	1 small	.24
Parsley	1/2 cup	5.50
Peanuts	1/2 cup	31.00
Peanut Oil	6 tablespoons	22.00
Peas, Green	1 cup	4.00
Potatoes, White	1 medium	.06
Potatoes, Sweet	1 small	4.00
Rice, Brown	3/4 cup cooked	2.40
Rye	1/2 cup	3.00
Soybean Oil	6 Tablespoons	140.00
Sunflower Seed	1/2 cup	31.00
Wheatgerm Oil (Crude)	6 tablespoons	150 - 420.00
Wheatgerm Oil (Medicinal)	6 tablespoons	320.00

When you're going to eat bread, be sure to buy only whole grain bread. Better yet, bake your own. I try to bake a delicious variety of breads once a week. Try our healthy recipes in Bragg's 448 page *Gourmet Recipe Book*. (See back pages for book list.)

Another rich food source of Vitamin E is cornmeal mush, made with organic stoneground yellow cornmeal (not the refined, dead, degerminated variety found in most commercial markets). Here is our favorite cornmeal recipe:

Patricia's Organic Cornmeal Mush

1 cup Organic Yellow Cornmeal
4 cups Distilled Water
3 Tbsp raisins (optional)

Thicken meal with 1/2 cup cold water. Boil balance of water, then slowly add the thickened cornmeal and raisins. Mix well. When evenly thickened, place in top of double boiler with heat turned very low, cook for 15 minutes (depending upon flavor desired).

Serve hot, top with honey or blackstrap molasses or 100% pure maple syrup (our favorite) and sliced fresh fruit (bananas are delicious).

NOTE: If you are serving this to only 1 or 2 people, there will be some mush left over. Pour it into a flat pan, let it cool and put it into the refrigerator. For breakfast – or even a main meal – slice and dip in egg batter and roll in wheatgerm. Saute in olive oil and serve hot topped with honey, blackstrap molasses or 100% pure maple syrup.

EAT FOR MORE SUPER OXYGEN, ENERGY AND HEALTH

Raw organic vegetables and fruits are Vitamin E rich and contain large amounts of oxygen. Their juices are especially rich in oxygen and distilled water – Nature's purest liquid!

Unsaturated oils – preferably cold or expeller pressed – are exceptionally rich in Vitamin E. Combine oil (canola, olive, safflower, soy) with lemon or orange juice or organic raw apple cider vinegar as a dressing for a combination vegetable salad. You will be eating both Vitamin E and oxygen.

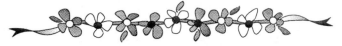

YOUR PULSE RATE MOST OFTEN REFLECTS YOUR FITNESS LEVEL
When you awaken in the morning – before moving – take your pulse for one full minute. This is your resting pulse. People with pulse rates from 40 to 60 are very fit, 60 to 80 are normal, and 80 to 100 are usually unfit.

Green leafy vegetables also supply organic iron and copper, vital minerals needed to manufacture hemoglobin in red blood cells. It enables the blood to absorb oxygen from the lungs and transport it to every part of the body.

Raw wheatgerm, besides supplying the body with Vitamin E, is also an important source of organic iron and copper. Other valuable sources for these minerals are blackberries, blackstrap molasses, dried unsulphured apricots, raw nuts and seeds, dandelion greens, dates, organ meats, such as liver, heart, sweetbreads and brains and also fertile egg yolks.

Some cooked foods enhance a naturally well balanced and nutritious diet. But cooking reduces and may eliminate the oxygen and vitamin content . . . don't overcook! We recommend that you steam, bake, broil, stir-fry or wok cook most foods.

The Bragg Healthy Lifestyle Promotes Super Health and Super Energy

When you eat according to the Bragg Healthy Lifestyle 60 to 65% of your diet will consist of fresh, live foods (organic is best), raw vegetables, salads, fresh fruits and juices, sprouts, raw seeds & nuts, plus natural 100% whole grain breads (preferably home baked), whole grain pastas & cereal, brown rice, & nutritious beans & legumes. You can make healthy and delicious combination salads, casseroles, soups, etc. and nutritious blender drinks people of all ages will love.

These are the no cholesterol, no fat, no salt *live foods* which provide body fuel for increased health and vitality. These foods make joyous, healthy, live energized people.

Following the Bragg Healthy Lifestyle you will become revitalized and reborn into a fresh new life filled with joy, vitality, youthfulness and longevity. There are millions of healthy Bragg followers around the world who have proved to themselves that the Bragg Healthy Lifestyle works miracles.

Discover hundreds of healthy and delicious recipes in our *Bragg's* 448 page *Complete Gourmet Health Recipes* and *The Vegetarian Cook Book and* you will never lack variety in your Bragg Healthy Lifestyle diet. (See back pages for Bragg Book info.)

Chapter 11

Health Schedule of 12 Meals Per Week

Natural nutrition and correct breathing habits together will lift you to higher levels of vibration for happy, healthful living. To attain and maintain the peak of Super Health, I practice and recommend eating two meals per day, with a pure distilled water fast for one 24 hour period each week.

Upon arising, before my Breathing Exercises, I drink the **Bragg Apple Cider Vinegar Cocktail: 1 to 2 tsp ACV plus 1 to 2 tsp raw honey in a glass of pure distilled water**. Read *The Miracles of Apple Cider Vinegar* for info on ACV.

After my breathing exercises I try to get from one to three hours of outdoor exercise: brisk walking, biking, swimming, hiking, weightlifting, gardening, etc. Then I have some fresh fruit or the Bragg Pep Drink, before I get to work writing, etc.

My first real meal comes about midday. This gives the stomach a thorough rest of 16 to 18 hours, allowing it time to completely empty, recuperate, and accumulate an abundant supply of digestive juices after the previous evening's meal.

Relax and chew your food thoroughly so the digestive process will get off to a good start and your food will be assimilated to give you the energy you need.

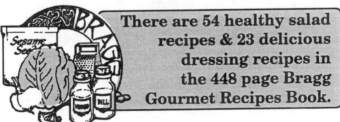

There are 54 healthy salad recipes & 23 delicious dressing recipes in the 448 page Bragg Gourmet Recipes Book.

The sense of obligation to continue is present in all of us. A duty to strive is the duty of us all. I felt a call to that duty. – Abraham Lincoln

LUNCH TIME IS SALAD POWER TIME

These days most people have work schedules which do not permit a rest after the midday meal. In Spain, Mexico, etc. the main meal is at midday and is followed by a siesta. This short nap is ideal, giving you two days in one. Rushed Americans eat their main meal in the evening and eat lightly at noon.

A full-meal salad of raw fruits or vegetables (organically grown when possible) with raw nuts, sunflower or sesame seeds or tofu cheese for protein makes a delicious and ideal luncheon. This is our favorite Bragg Salad recipe:

BRAGG FAMOUS RAW VEGETABLE GARDEN SALAD

2 *stalks celery, sliced*
1/4 *diced bellpepper & seeds*
1/4 *cucumber, sliced*
3 *medium tomatoes*
2 *spring onions with tops*
1/2 *cup green cabbage, sliced*

1/3 *cup red cabbage, chopped*
1/2 *C alfalfa or sunflower sprouts*
1 *raw beet, grated*
1 *carrot, grated*
1 *turnip, grated*
1 *avocado (ripe)*

For variety add raw zucchini, cauliflower, mushrooms, broccoli or sugar peas. Chop, slice or grate vegetables medium to fine for variety in size. Mix vegetables thoroughly and serve on a bed of lettuce, spinach, watercress or chopped cabbage. Dice avocado & tomato, & serve on side as a dressing. Serve choice of fresh squeezed lemon, orange or dressing separately. Chill salad plates in freezer before using. Always eat your salad first before serving hot dishes. Serves 3 to 5.

DELICIOUS BRAGG VINAIGRETTE HEALTH DRESSING

1 *tsp fresh herbs, minced, or pinch Italian dry herbs*
1 to 2 *tsp raw honey*   1 to 2 *cloves garlic, minced*
1/2 *C Bragg Organic Raw Apple Cider Vinegar*
1/3 *tsp Bragg Liquid Aminos*
blend with 1/3 *C Virgin Olive Oil*

Combine ingredients in jar and refrigerate.

HONEY VINAIGRETTE CELERY SEED DRESSING

1/4 *tsp dry mustard*
1/4 *tsp Bragg Liquid Aminos*
1/4 *tsp paprika*
2 *Tbsp raw honey*

1/2 *C Bragg Apple Cider Vinegar*
2 *Tbsp virgin olive oil*
1 *small onion, minced*
1/4 *tsp celery seed*

Blend ingredients in blender or jar, then last add onion and celery seed and blend lightly. Refrigerate in covered jar.

For delicious herbal or fruit vinegars: in quart jar add 1/2 cup tightly packed fruit or crushed fresh sweet basil, tarragon, dill, oregano, or any fresh herbs desired, combined or singly. (If *dried* herbs, use 1 to 2 tsp herbs.) Add Bragg Raw Apple Cider Vinegar, store 2 weeks in warm place, then strain and refrigerate.

ENJOY HEALTHY, BALANCED VARIETY FOR DINNER

Relax at day's end with some Super Power Breaths. Clean the day's toxins from your lungs so that you will get the full benefit from a well-balanced, nourishing and tasteful dinner! Your basic health menu should include:

Salad . . . a smaller serving this time of fresh raw vegetables and/or fruits. Try these suggestions: grated cabbage with diced bell peppers and grated carrots . . . or grated carrots with fresh sliced apple or pineapple and raisins . . . or lettuce, tomato and cucumber salad. Make salad dressing of olive oil and natural apple cider vinegar or lemon or orange juice. Sprinkle with wheatgerm, nutritional yeast (flakes) or Parmesan cheese for added zest.

Cooked Vegetables . . . include one green and one yellow vegetable, lightly cooked, steamed, baked or stir-fried. *Never add salt!* Season with Bragg Liquid Aminos for taste delights.

Protein Dish . . . may be either vegetable or animal. Vegetable proteins include all beans, brown rice, lentils, tofu. etc. and all raw, unsalted nuts and seeds (sunflower, pumpkin, sesame, etc.). We prefer a vegetarian diet, but if you eat meat, do so no more than 3 times a week. Meat should be skinless chicken or turkey, lean lamb or beef, liver, fish (from unpolluted waters). Never add table salt. Prepare your foods with healthy, nutritious additions: fresh garlic, onions, lemon juice, herbs and add delicious Bragg Liquid Aminos (made from soy beans).

Dessert . . . if eaten, should be fresh fruit or, if unavailable, unsweetened or honey-stewed fruit. For special treats try the healthy pies, cakes, cookies, etc. in the Bragg Recipe Books.

Beverages . . . for Super-Health, do not drink beverages with your meals . . . not even water! Let your digestive juices do their work undiluted. Be sure to have ample fluids in the daytime, and then an hour after dinner, have the delicious Bragg Vinegar Drink (hot or cold), herb tea, or a glass of fruit or vegetable juice, if you wish. Drink all the water, preferably distilled, that you want between meals.

DO NOT POISON YOUR BODY
WITH FOODLESS FOODS AND HARMFUL DRINKS

In our industrialized, urbanized civilization, we pay a heavy price for the convenience of mass distribution of foodstuffs. Not only has our flour been bleached and robbed of its vital wheatgerm, but the majority of commercialized foods have been devitalized, demineralized–rendered *foodless* –in order to give them a longer *shelf life.* You are risking your own life to eat these *foodless* foods that cannot nourish your body properly. Many contain preservative *additives* (such as nitrates and nitrites) whose cumulative effect has proven to be extremely harmful to the human body.

Although the FDA (Federal Food and Drug Administration) tries to protect the consumer by requiring the listing of most ingredients on processed, packaged and canned foods, few people bother to read the fine print. If they do, they rarely understand what they read or take the trouble to find out what the various additives are and what effect they have on the human body. You don't have to be a chemist to find the answers; all you have to do is to use a modern dictionary.

For example, Webster's Collegiate Dictionary defines *nitrate* as *a salt or ester of nitric acid* . . . and defines *nitric acid* as *a corrosive liquid inorganic acid* HNO_3 . Now, it doesn't require more than ordinary commonsense to figure out what a steady diet of foods containing a concentrated form of a corrosive liquid inorganic acid is going to do to your body!

Sulphur dioxide is another commercial preservative, used commonly on dried fruits. It is defined by Webster as *a heavy pungent gas, easily condensed to a colorless liquid and used especially in making sulfuric acid.* Do I have to remind you that sulfuric acid eats away flesh?

Many natural fats are ruined by *hydrogenation,* a hardening process which keeps them from becoming rancid but renders them absolutely indigestible and cardiovascular cloggers.

Read those labels and understand them. Eliminate from your diet all commercially refined and processed foods: refined white flour, refined white sugar and products made with these, processed *lunch meats* and cheeses, hydrogenated fats, foods with harmful preservatives or additives such as monosodium glutamate, sodium nitrate, sulfur dioxide, etc.

Although these are not labeled *poison*, banish from your diet coffee, tea and alcohol, all of which contain harmful

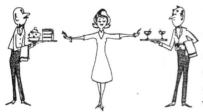

ingredients that become cumulative poisons in your body. Also avoid soft drinks and cola drinks which contain nothing but *empty calories* that will toxify your vital bloodstream and body.

DO NOT USE TABLE SALT!

Salt was the first food preservative discovered by man. It has been used for so many thousands of years that countless generations of *civilized* humans have believed salt to be a necessity of life. Primitive peoples know better. They don't use added salt in their native diets. They remain remarkably healthy, until they are discovered by civilized men and introduced to the poisons of civilization. Then their deterioration is rapid and tragic. I have seen this happen in the South Sea Islands, in Africa and in the Arctic.

We cannot stress it often enough: Never use table salt!

The *salt of the earth* (inorganic sodium chloride) is poor food for plants and poison for animals, including man. What about *salt licks*? Don't even wild animals *lick salt*? My father investigated this thoroughly – and found that **natural salt licks never contain sodium chloride, but are made up of organic minerals from decomposed plant life.** We regret to report that the commercial salt licks used by cattle ranchers are for the purpose of making the cattle thirsty so that they will drink great volumes of water, and therefore weigh more when they are ready to be sold. This is why meat so often *shrinks* excessively when you cook it.

All animals, including man, need organic minerals. Only plants can digest inorganic minerals, which they take from the earth and convert through photosynthesis into organic minerals to feed the animal kingdom. This is Mother Nature's marvelous balance.

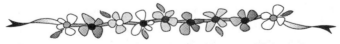

Everything in excess is opposed by Nature. – Hippocrates

When our ancestors discovered that salt, (inorganic sodium chloride), would preserve meat from decay, they had no refrigeration or means of storing food for long periods. Because their lifestyles were extremely active, their bodies were able to eliminate this indigestible inorganic mineral.

Civilized people today are usually a sedentary creatures. They cannot eliminate or assimilate the excessive amount of salt which they consume. Their bodies stash it away in crystals that harden the lining of the arteries, and other blood vessels, in joints causing arthritis and other pains and in water solution that bloats the tissues and can ultimately cause congestive heart failure.

Eliminate salt from your diet! If you think your food tastes *flat* without it, add Bragg Liquid Aminos, a delicious seasoning, or powdered sea kelp, which has a tangy taste. Or take a lesson from famous French chefs, who use very little or no salt, but achieve their marvelous flavors by the skillful use of onions, garlic, mushrooms and herbs. Lemon juice is good for seasoning salads. veggies, meat and fish.

Salt actually deadens your taste buds. Without it, your taste buds will awaken and you will enjoy the true, natural flavors of the food you eat. Even more importantly, you will feel better – and live longer, when you give up salt!

FAST ONE DAY EACH WEEK FOR INNER CLEANSING

Oxygen, as I have stressed, is the greatest cleanser and purifier of the body. Give it a chance to do a thorough house cleansing, to help the body rid itself of accumulated toxic poisons, by going on a 24 to 36 hour fast every week.

During this fast, drink six to eight glasses of distilled water daily, flavored with fresh lemon juice or 1 tsp of raw, organic apple cider vinegar with 1 tsp of honey, if you desire. . . and nothing else! No food, juices or supplements are necessary. If you feel the need to have something warm inside, have some herb tea or warm Bragg Apple Cider Vinegar Health Cocktail.

Freed from the daily chore of digesting and assimilating food, your body will use its oxygen-given energy to do a more thorough cleanse. After your first fast you will feel a renewed vitality. As you make this a weekly habit, and, as time goes on, you will feel even more invigorated and rejuvenated.

I take my regular weekly fast from Sunday evening to Tuesday morning. After my evening meal on Sunday, I take nothing but 6 to 8 glasses of distilled water until breakfast on Tuesday. We have been doing this fast in the Bragg family for the last 90 years and we are all living healthy, long lives. I always try to fast for the first three days of the month also.

Several times each year I take a longer *super* fast. My favorite is distilled water for an entire week . It works wonders in keeping me fit and trim. If you would like to know more about the methods and benefits of scientific fasting, consult our Bragg book, *The Miracle of Fasting.* (See back pages for book information.)

DISTILLED WATER IS THE #1 HEALTH DRINK

Not merely on your fast days, but every day of your life, let your drinking water be pure distilled water. You will be *drinking oxygen* with this pure H_2O. In addition to fresh fruit and vegetable juices . . . which are naturally distilled . . . this is the only *safe* water to drink on this polluted planet of ours.

Even rain water – which is naturally distilled water when it leaves the clouds – is contaminated if it passes through a heavily polluted atmosphere. (I love the smell of rain washed air.)

Mineral water and ground water (from springs, wells, streams, etc.) usually contain inorganic minerals which are not assimilated by the body and which can produce harmful deposits in the blood vessels, joints, kidneys and gallbladder.

Water from reservoirs, which has been chemically treated to kill germs, contains inorganic minerals, as well as harsh chemicals, such as chlorine which are extremely harmful to the body! Do not drink water produced by water softeners. It contains suspended inorganic minerals that produce more *suds* in the water, but this water is harmful to your body.

Use distilled water for drinking and cooking to insure long life and health for you and your family! You will find the complete, documented report on the health hazards of ordinary water and the reasons for drinking only distilled water in our book, *The Shocking Truth About Water!* (See back pages for info.)

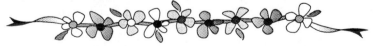

Now learn what great benefits a temperate diet will bring with it.
In the first place you enjoy good health. – Horace, 65 B.C.

AVOID THESE PROCESSED, REFINED, HARMFUL FOODS

Once you realize the irreparable harm caused to your body by refined, chemicalized, deficient foods, it is easy to eat correctly. Simply eliminate these "killer" foods from your diet and follow the Bragg Healthy Lifestyle. It provides the basic, essential nourishment your body needs to maintain you in super energy and health.

• Refined sugar or refined sugar products such as jams, jellies, preserves, marmalades, yogurts, ice cream, sherberts, Jello, cake, candy, cookies, chewing gum, soft drinks, pies, pastries, tapioca puddings, sugared fruit, juices & fruits canned in sugar syrup.

• Salted foods, such as corn chips, salted crackers, salted nuts.

• White rice & pearled barley.   • Fried & greasy foods.

• Commercial, highly processed dry cereals such as corn flakes, etc.

• Saturated fats & hydrogenated oils – enemies that clog bloodstream.

• Food which contains palm & cottonseed oil. Products labeled vegetable oil . . . find out what kind before you use it.

• Oleo & margarine . . . (saturated fats & hydrogenated oils).

• Peanut butter that contains hydrogenated, hardened oils.

• Coffee, decaffeinated coffee, China black tea & all alcoholic beverages.

• Fresh pork & pork products.   • Fried, fatty & greasy meats.

• Smoked meats, such as ham, bacon, sausage & smoked fish.

• Luncheon meats, hot dogs, salami, bologna, corned beef, pastrami & packaged meats containing dangerous sodium nitrate or nitrite.

• Dried fruits containing sulphur dioxide - a preservative.

• Do not eat chickens or turkeys that have been injected with stilbestrol, or fed with poultry feed that contains any drugs.

• Canned soups - read labels for sugar, starch, flour & preservatives.

• Food that contains benzoate of soda, salt, sugar, cream of tartar & any additives, drugs or preservatives.

• White flour products such as white bread, wheat-white bread, enriched flours, rye bread that has wheat-flour in it, dumplings, biscuits, buns, gravy, noodles, pancakes, waffles, soda crackers, macaroni, spaghetti, pizza, ravioli, pies, pastries, cakes, cookies, prepared and commercial puddings and ready-mix bakery products. (Health Food Stores have huge varieties of 100% whole grain products – breads, crackers, pastas, pastries, etc.).

• Day-old cooked vegetables & potatoes & old pre-mi

• Pasteurized & filtered vinegars, malt & synthetic vinegars & distilled white vinegar. These are dead vinegars! *For info read Bragg Vinegar Book.*
(We use only organic, raw unfiltered Apple Cider Vinegar.)

Chapter 12

A Strong Mind In A Strong Body

Greek civilization, which produced some of the greatest minds the world has known, lived by the motto: *A strong mind in a strong body.* Ancient Greeks were noted for their amazing powers of endurance and healthy longevity, as well as their system of eating, deep breathing and exercising which produced physiques that have been models of art ever since.

The Greek System followed three main health principles:

1. Full, deep breathing.

2. Eating natural foods on the 2-meals-per-day schedule.

3. Systematized exercise for complete body development.

We can do the same and achieve the same results they did. We can become vital and totally fit – enjoying every minute of being alive. The time to start is NOW . . . whatever your calendar years. Whether you are a teenager or a great-grandparent or somewhere in between, it is never too early or too late to start on the Road to Super-Health!

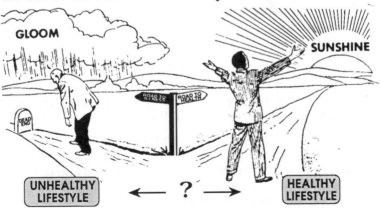

The choice of which road to take is up to the individual. He alone can decide whether he wants to reach a dead end or live a healthy lifestyle for a long, happy, active life. — Paul C. Bragg

SUPER-OXYGEN BREATHING FOR SUPER-LIVING

When your body is fed with Live Foods and Super Oxygen, the joy of living will thrill you. Every day you bounce out of bed with a *glad to be alive* feeling knowing there is meaning in life. You have no depressed thoughts, no *down in the mouth* feeling, no envy, no hatreds, no jealousies, no blue Mondays, no frustrations, no fears, worries, anxieties, no morbid feelings.

With the stimulation of Super Oxygen, you are eager to meet life's problems. You meet them face to face and find solutions. You enjoy the effort of facing life's realities. You use fully the intelligence and commonsense God gave you. Those people who know how to breathe deeply do not run away from life, but face it with courage and determination. The weakling, inevitably a shallow breather, takes the escape route: alcohol, drugs and self-pity that can lead to illness.

THE ADVANTAGES OF SUPER POWER BREATHING

1. The most important of all physical acts is correct breathing. No one can be perfectly well and healthy who does not breathe deeply. Super Power Breathing Exercises help you to create the habit of correct breathing at all times.

2. When you breathe correctly, you add millions of health-giving, oxygen-carrying red blood cells to your bloodstream.

3. When you fill the entire lungs with oxygen, you cleanse your body of toxic poisons that could do you great damage.

4. When sufficient oxygen is taken into the system, you will no longer crave artificial stimulants. Oxygen is the only stimulation that has no harmful after-affects.

5. When more oxygen gets into your bloodstream, you will feel Super Energized and will have greater health!

6. Super Power Deep Breathing is now a part of every cure. Today, in the modern hospital, pure oxygen often heals when every other method of healing has failed. Even broken bones heal more quickly when the blood is purified by doing daily Deep Breathing Exercises.

7. Deep Breathing is the great body normalizer. Oxygen is the invisible food for the body and helps with assimilation of your foods. Deep Breathing Exercises will also help people attain and maintain a more normal, healthy weight.

8. *Super Power Breathing helps make the weak strong, and athletes champions.* – Bob Anderson, trainer of champions

9. Many nervous diseases are due to oxygen starvation. Deep, diaphragmatic breathing tranquilizes jangled nerves and stimulates the brain to alertness and profound thought.

10. If everyone understood and practiced Super Power Breathing, there would be no need for eye, ear, nose and throat specialists. The oxygen filling these cavities destroys germs lodged there, and creates healthy circulation in these areas.

11. Many people suffer from poor circulation in various parts of the body. Because they don't get sufficient oxygen to produce a steady circulation of the blood into their extremities, they have cold hands, feet, noses and ears. The more oxygen you get into you, the better the circulation in your system is.

12. People who get sufficient oxygen have better muscle tone. Their skin is healthier, firmer and more alive.

13. Oxygen is Nature's great beautifier. It gives the skin a radiant glow and the hair a lustrous sheen.

14. People who breathe in large amounts of oxygen are happier people. Deep breathing cleanses your body of psychological and physical poisons and gives you more joy for your daily living and emotional well being.

15. Digestive ills are often eliminated by the internal massage of correct diaphragmatic action. Every time a Power Breath is taken, the digestive tract is gently exercised.

16. Slow, deep breaths soothe and recharge the heart. Conversely, rapid, shallow breathing exhausts it through overwork and lack of sufficient oxygen for the blood.

17. Probably the last thing one would expect to be influenced by correct breathing is straightening of the teeth. Yet much corrective work of the best American dental colleges consists of deep diaphragmatic breathing. Correct breathing normalizes the cavities of the nose, mouth and throat, and exerts a gentle pressure upon the teeth.

18. Oxygen, the great invisible food, stimulant and purifier, builds our resistance to infections and strengthens our weak points. It's Nature's most vital aid in helping the body to heal itself and to stay healthy. Better the ounce of prevention than the pound of cure! **Start now to Breathe fully and live fully!**

These freshly squeezed vegetable and fruit juices are important to the Bragg Healthy Lifestyle. We feel it's not wise to drink beverages with your main meals. But if during the day you wish a glass of freshly squeezed orange, grapefruit, vegetable juice, Bragg Vinegar Drink, herb tea or try a hot cup of Bragg Liquid Aminos Broth (1/2 to 1 tsp Bragg Liquid Aminos in cup of hot distilled water) . . . these are all ideal pick-me-up beverages.

The Bragg Favorite Juice Cocktail – This drink consists of all raw vegetables (please – organic when possible) which we prepare in our vegetable juicer: Carrots, Celery, Beets, Cabbage, Watercress and Parsley. The great purifier Garlic is optional.

The Bragg Favorite Health "Pep" Drink – After our morning exercises often we enjoy this instead of fruit. It's also delicious and powerfully nutritious as a meal anytime: lunch, dinner or to take in a thermos to work, school, to the park or hiking, etc.

BRAGG HEALTHY PEP DRINK

Prepare the following in blender, add 1 ice cube if desired colder:

Choice of: freshly squeezed orange juice; carrot and greens juice; unsweetened pineapple juice; or 1-1/2 cups distilled water with:

1/2 tsp raw wheatgerm	1/4 tsp Vitamin C powder
1/3 tsp flax seed oil, optional	1/4 tsp nutritional yeast flakes
1/4 tsp green powder (barley, etc.)	1 to 2 bananas, ripe
1/2 tsp raw oat bran	1 tsp raw honey, optional
1/2 tsp psyllium husk powder	1 tsp soy protein powder
1/2 tsp lecithin granules	1 tsp raw sunflower seeds

Optional: 4 apricots (sundried, unsulphured). Soak in jar overnight in distilled water or unsweetened pineapple juice. We soak enough to last for several days. Keep refrigerated. In summer you can add fresh fruit in season: peaches, strawberries, berries, apricots, etc. instead of the banana. In winter add apples, oranges, pears or persimmons or try sugar-free, frozen fruits. Serves 1 to 2.

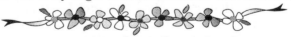

Patricia's Delicious Health Popcorn

Use freshly popped popcorn (my favorite is the non-oil, air popped). If desired, use olive, soy, or canola oil, or melted salt-free butter. Add several dashes or sprays of Bragg's Liquid Aminos to the oil and pour over popcorn. Sprinkle with nutritional yeast flakes or grated Parmesan cheese. For variety, add a pinch of Italian herbs, cayenne pepper, mustard powder or fresh crushed garlic to the liquid mixture.

Chapter 13

DOCTOR FRESH AIR

Dr. Fresh Air is a specialist, and his greatest prescription is *The Breath of God's Pure Fresh Air, the invisible staff of life.*

The first thing we do when we are born is to take a long, deep breath and the final thing we do is take a last gasp, before we stop breathing. Between birth and death, our life is completely maintained by our breathing.

Dr. Fresh Air wants you to have a long, healthy life. Practice these simple deep breathing exercises and remain conscious that with every breath you take you are bringing into your body the breath of God, the life-giving oxygen.

People who fail to obey the doctor's orders about getting plenty of fresh air day and night invite extremely severe complications. Let us examine very closely the function of breathing. It is invisible food – the only food that we absolutely cannot live without. If we are deprived of air for over five to seven minutes death will take us. We are breathing machines.

Air supplies us with life-giving oxygen which is critical for every cell in our bodies. Oxygen is carried by the blood to the lungs where a great miracle takes place: life-giving oxygen is exchanged for deadly carbon dioxide. We create deadly toxins in the process of living that CO_2 carries out of our bodies. These are collected by the blood, brought to our lungs and expelled as the new life-giving oxygen enters. During the process of metabolism, in the building up and tearing down of the cells of the body, carbon dioxide poison is constantly burned up in the very process of living.

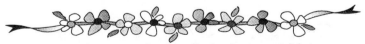

Now I see the secret of making the best persons. It is to grow in the open air, and eat and sleep with the earth. – Walt Whitman

When a person does not get enough fresh air, or is a shallow breather, and the intake of oxygen does not equal the output of carbon dioxide, then this poison can build up in the body. This could result in serious physical problems because the retained carbon dioxide can be concentrated in some other parts of the body and could cause intense physical problems and suffering.

Enervation, or the lack of nerve energy, can lower the Vital Force so much that the lungs, cannot pump in enough air to flush carbon dioxide out of the body. You can see how important it is that you breathe fresh air, and you must always be conscious of the fact that you must breathe deeply.

We are air machines. Miracle oxygen purifies our bodies. It's one of the great energizers of the human body. We are air-pressure machines. We live at the bottom of an atmospheric ocean approximately 70 miles deep. This air pressure is 14 pounds per square inch. Between the inhalation and the exhalation of a breath, a vacuum is formed. As long as we continue to have this rhythmical intake and outgo of oxygen, we will live. We know that we can go without food for 30 days or more and still survive, but we can only go without air for a very few minutes. Air is one of the most important energizers of the human body. The more deeply you breathe pure air, the better your chances are for extending your years on this earth.

For over 70 years, my father did extensive research on long-lived people and found one common denominator among all of them: they are deep breathers! The deeper, therefore fewer breaths a person takes in one minute, the longer that person lives. Rapid breathers are short-lived people. This also holds true in the animal world. Rabbits, guinea pigs, and all kinds of rodents are rapid breathers, taking many breaths every minute. They are the shortest-lived breathing creatures on the face of the earth. For years I have made it a practice when I first get up in the morning to take long, slow, deep breaths. During the day, I also try to take periods where I breathe long, deeper full breaths. Try this, it's wonderful!

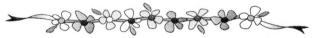

Enthusiasm is the vital quality that arouses and inspires you to action.
– Paul C. Bragg

INDIA HOLY MEN PRACTICE DEEP, SLOW BREATHING

In my father's expeditions into India, he found holy men in secluded retreats who devoted their lives to building a physically powerful body as an instrument for high spiritual advancement. They spend many hours daily in the practice of rhythmic, long, slow, deep breaths. These holy men of India were utterly fantastic physically. The deep breathing of fresh air kept their skin and muscle-tone ageless. He met a holy man in the foothills of the Himalaya Mountains who told him that he was, at that time, 126 years old. This man had no reason to lie to him, because his whole life was spent in getting closer to God. It was he who taught my father the system which we expanded upon and now teach all over the world as *Bragg Super Power Breathing*.

This holy man had perfect vision, and he had a beautiful head of hair. He had all his teeth and the endurance and stamina of an athlete. He spoke five languages fluently. He was one of the most amazing men my father ever met! When asked to what he owed his great strength and mentality, he answered, *I have made a long life practice of breathing deeply and practicing faithfully all of my breathing meditations daily.*

My father did not like to guess the age of any person, but while he was on this trip to India, he met a woman, whose age he guessed to be about 50. He was amazed when she told him she was 86. She was a beautiful woman with virtually no sign of deterioration, and he asked her the secret of her beauty and her agelessness. Again he got the same answer he did from the holy man – this beautiful woman was conscious of the importance of deep, slow breathing.

UNCOMPLICATE YOUR LIVING

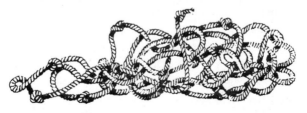

Meditation is easy – we complicate it. – J Krishnamurti

No doubt, you have noticed rosy-cheeked children running and playing, jumping rope, roller-skating and bicycling. While they are doing these activities, they are breathing in large amounts of oxygen, and that is what we must keep in mind. We must keep active. We must take long, brisk walks and cultivate the habit of slow, deep breathing. When people live sedentary, uncreative lives and no longer get vigorous exercise, they are harming and shortening their lives.

SUPER POWER DEEP BREATHING: THE SECRET OF ENDURANCE AND STAMINA

We had a long time friend named Amos Stagg, the famous California football and athletic coach. Mr. Stagg lived over 100 active, happy years. I asked him his secret of long life at his 100th birthday party. His answer was, *I have the greater part of my life indulged in running and other vigorous exercise that forced large amounts of oxygen into my body and this along with working with athletes has kept me youthful.*

Dad had a friend in New York, James Hocking, who was one of the greatest long distance walking champions this country has ever had. I asked Mr. Hocking, on his hundredth birthday, the secret of his long, active life and super health. His answer was, *I have always walked vigorously and breathed deeply.* As you can see, oxygen is a detoxifier. It is a cleansing miracle. Like fasting, it helps remove toxins from the body.

I practice deep breathing and believe people should expose their bodies to a free current of moving air. Air baths are important for good health. Whenever possible sleep with your windows wide open with cross ventilated air moving across your body. I sleep better and have a deeper night's rest, if I wear light sleeping garments of cotton or silk, or nothing at all. You will be warm under the covers. But if you sleep with heavy blankets and nightwear, you smother your skin's vital oxygen supply and increase your chance of illness.

You must compensate for the hours you spend sitting down, because it inhibits your natural, healthy breathing. If your work requires a lot of sitting, you should compensate for it with outdoor walking and physical activities.

You will find that you can solve most of your problems on a brisk one to three mile hike. Whenever I have a problem to solve, I always take a long brisk walk in the fresh air. By the time I have finished my walk, I have found a solution. I believe that after the evening meal, everyone should make a practice of taking a leisurely walk (arms swinging) – even if it has to be up and down their driveway. Today people have become sitters. They sit at their desks, at movies, concerts, while watching athletics and television. They are air-starved, oxygen-starved and exercise-starved.

When we cannot get the carbon dioxide out of our bodies, we develop aches, pains and become prone to premature ageing. This is all because we are indifferent about being active people. On any city street, you can see pale, ghostly people, unhealthy and exhausted – mostly as a result of air-starvation.

It is critical to fast also, because it enables you to clean some of this concentrated, stored-up carbon dioxide that failed to leave your body by deep breathing. When you are fasting, enjoy walking – even if it is a short one. Make it a regular part of your life to be an active person. That does not mean house-walks. It means getting out in the fresh air hiking, biking, running, swimming, or dancing, etc. You must not allow any carbon dioxide to build up in your body, it will only bring about serious health consequences.

Make it a point every day of your life to breathe deeply during a vigorous brisk walk – or some other aerobic exercise. **Take long, slow, deep breaths every time you think of it.** Soon your slow, deep breathing becomes a normal habit. When you combine deep breathing with fasting and living the Bragg Healthy Lifestyle, you are building more health, energy and vitality and you will live longer. Remind yourself every day that Doctor Fresh Air is your constant friend!

Live with enthusiasm and your days and life will be filled with more joy, health and happiness! – Patricia Bragg

---

Carbon Dioxide (CO2) in soda drinks causes the lungs to have to work harder to eliminate the excess waste product. – Basic Physiology

---

Ninety percent of our metabolic oxygen comes from breathing. Ten percent comes from food. – Dr. Gabriel Cousins

---

Nerve force contains much of its power in the breath. – Yoga Sutras

Exercise and Eat for Health and Longevity

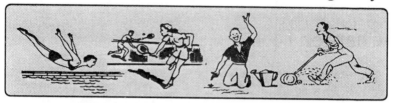

BRAGG HEALTHY LIFESTYLE
FOR A LIFETIME OF SUPER HEALTH

In a broad sense, "The Bragg Healthy Lifestyle for the Total Person" is a combination of physical, mental, emotional, social and spiritual components. The ability of the individual to function effectively in his environment depends on how smoothly these components function as a whole. Of all the qualities that comprise an integrated personality, a totally healthy, fit body is one of the most desirable . . . so start today for achieving your health goals!

A person may be said to be totally physically fit if he functions as a total personality with efficiency and without pain or discomfort of any kind. This is to have a Painless, Tireless, Ageless body, possessing sufficient muscular strength and endurance to maintain a healthy posture and successfully carry on the duties imposed by life and the environment, to meet emergencies satisfactorily and have enough energy for recreation and social obligations after the "work day" has ended. It is to meet the requirements for his environment through possessing the resilience to recover rapidly from fatigue, tension, stress and strain of daily living without the aid of stimulants, drugs or alcohol, and enjoy natural recharging sleep at night and awaken fit and alert in the morning for the challenges of the new fresh day ahead.

Keeping the body totally healthy and fit is not a job for the uninformed or the careless person. It requires an understanding of the body and of a healthy lifestyle and then following that lifestyle for a long, happy life. The result of the "Bragg Healthy Lifestyle" is to wake up the possibilities within you, rejuvenate your body, mind and soul to total balanced health . . . . It's within your reach, so don't procrastinate, start today! Our hearts go out to touch your heart with nourishing, caring love for your total health.

Patricia Bragg and Paul C. Bragg

Dear friend, I wish above all things that thou may prosper and be in health even as the soul prospers. – 3 John 2

80

Chapter 14

DOCTOR REST

Dr. Rest is another specialist always at your command to help you achieve Supreme Vitality. I believe the word *rest* is the most misunderstood word in the English language. Some people's idea of resting is to sit down and drink a cup of strong stimulant, such as coffee, black tea or caffeinated soft drinks. This is typified by the *coffee break*. To me, rest means repose, freedom from activity, quiet, tranquility. It means peace of mind and spirit, it means to rest without anxiety or worry, and it means to refresh one's self. Your rest should refresh your whole nervous system and your entire body.

When you are resting, you cannot sit with one leg crossed over the other, because this position puts a tremendous burden on the artery which supplies the feet with blood and also cuts off nerve energy. If you sit with your legs crossed, you are not resting, but giving the heart a tremendous load of work to do. When you sit down – keep both feet on the floor.

To rest means to allow a free circulation (no restrictions) of blood throughout the entire body. If your shoes are too tight, if your collar is too tight, if your hat is too tight, if your belt or any of your undergarments are too tight, if stockings are too tight, you are not resting when you sit still or lie down.

Why do we rest? Often people say, I *need to rest!* But when they sit down intending to rest, they nervously drum their fingers on a table or desk, or they squirm and move restlessly.

The art of resting is something that must be acquired and concentrated upon. The best rest is secured when your body is freed from restrictive clothing. Any clothes you are wearing should be comfortably loose and never binding.

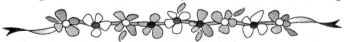

I cannot overstate the importance of the habit of quiet meditation and prayer for more health of body, mind and spirit. – Patricia Bragg

One good way to rest is to lie down on a firm bed or couch unclothed or with as few loose clothes as possible. Another good way to rest is to sunbathe. There is nothing that will relax the muscles and nerves like the gentle, soothing rays of the sun. In order to rest, you must learn to clear your mind of all anxiety, worries and emotional problems. When the muscles and nerves are relaxed, the heart action slows – especially when you take long, slow, deep breaths. This will bring deep relaxation and more total rest.

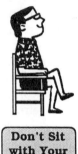

Don't Sit with Your Legs Crossed – It Hinders Circulation

CHECK YOUR MATTRESS

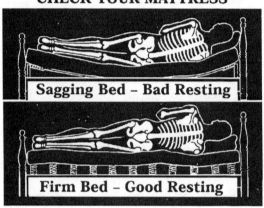

Sagging Bed – Bad Resting

Firm Bed – Good Resting

ENJOY RELAXATION – IT'S NO CRIME

Another good form of resting is a short nap. When you take a nap, command your muscles to become completely relaxed. Your conscious and subconscious mind controls the muscles and the nerves, so you must be in complete command of your body when you rest. The Master Teacher and His Disciples, when worn and weary, said, *Come Ye and Rest a While.* The Master did not lead them into the busy streets of Jerusalem where there was noise and clatter. He didn't even take them into the synagogue. He took them into the quiet of the wide open spaces, under the blue sky. Here, He could rebuild, relax and revive every organ of their exhausted bodies and revitalize, refresh and invigorate their weary minds. The greatest place to rest, relax, and renew your Vital Force is under the blue sky in the clean, fresh air. On hot days enjoy the shade of trees.

Sleep is the greatest revitalizer we have, but few people get a long, peaceful and refreshing night's sleep. Most people habitually use stimulants: tobacco, drugs, coffee, tea, and other caffeinated drinks which whip tired nerves. People who use these stimulants never have complete rest and relaxation because their nerves are always in an excited condition.

Most people do not earn their rest. Rest must be earned with physical and mental activity, because they go hand in hand. So many people complain what poor sleepers they are – that they toss and turn throughout the night. For an extra relaxer before bedtime try our Bragg Apple Cider Vinegar Cocktail hot or cold (It's delicious, see recipe on page 63).

Today, millions of people take some type of drug to induce sleep, but this is not true sleep. No one gets restful sleep with a sleeping tablets. You may drug yourself to unconsciousness, but that very drug will deprive you of a normal, restful, healthful and satisfying sleep.

When you do not eliminate the toxins from your body – your nerves are continually irritated. How is it possible to get a good night's rest with irritated nerves? When we live a healthy lifestyle, exercise, breathe deeply and perform our weekly 24 hour fast, we become restful sleepers. With fasting, we have discovered that when people discard their stimulants on a fasting program, they become deep, restful sleepers.

You will notice as you purify your body that you will be able to relax more readily. You will be able to enjoy naps, and you will enjoy the benefits of a long, restful, night's sleep. Rest is important! The Bible tells us that God appointed one day of rest every week for man. In this wonderful law, we have plentiful support for our contention that frequent change of activity is an important factor in the maintenance of super-health. To complement our busy days, we require the variety of recreational activities. The old adage is true, *All work and no play does make Jack a dull boy.*

Today we live in a hectic, competitive world, which in business parlance is called the *rat race.* During these stressful times, filled with political and emotional unrest we build up tremendous pressures, tensions and strains. This is why people turn to tobacco, drugs, coffee, alcohol and other harmful substances – to try to escape the stress.

There is not only competition in the business world, but in the social realm as well – as people strive to maintain their *status*. People are always trying to impress one another, and trying to create a certain *image*. They create a false image and it takes tremendous energy to portray this falseness! There is tremendous pressure on women who believe their worth is dependent on their appearance. So they spend hours having their hair colored, constantly trying to keep up with the latest fashions, struggling to have a different – perfect – body. All of this calls for energy. Our modern civilization drives and pushes us, robbing us of our natural, peaceful state.

LIFE IS TO BE SAVORED AND ENJOYED

It is no wonder that we have created millions of chronic alcoholics and drug addicts. Why have people completely forgotten that life is to be lived and enjoyed? Few in our society enjoy leisure living. Life is rush, rush, rush! Where are we rushing to? To the hospital or the graveyard?

To be able to relax, rest and sleep, you must program your day so you have time for work, rest, recreation, exercise and a good night's sleep. You cannot get a good night's sleep if you overload your stomach. You cannot have a good night's sleep unless you have earned it with outdoor exercise, such as a brisk, one to three mile walk or garden work, etc. Housework or your job are not the way to get exercise and activity. Here's a guide to help you. Let your body be nourished by healthy, natural food, pure distilled water, and plenty of fresh air and gentle sunlight. Enjoy a balanced program of exercise and repose and let Nature do the rest! Treat yourself as you deserve and the results will astound you! We, the *Back to Nature* people, have been ridiculed for years as faddists and extremists, but now our healthy lifestyle is in demand. The popular press daily has stories confirming what we have always known. We who believe in Mother Nature and God want to spread health, love, peace and happiness worldwide.

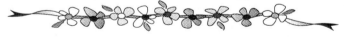

People who say it can't be done shouldn't interrupt those who are doing it.

Indians and animals know better how to live than white man; nobody can be in good health, if he does not have all the time fresh air, sunshine and good water. – Flying Hawk

LOVE MOTHER NATURE AND YOURSELF DAILY

We recommend that you slowly return to a more natural way of living, in food, clothing, rest, and in simplicity in living habits – strive for harmony with Mother Nature and God.

Live as Mother Nature wants. Realize that she loves you and you are part of her family. Put yourself in her hands and let her inner wisdom guide you. Mother Nature is eager to inspire and guide you, so she can help you tune up your human machine. She can help cleanse and repair it, if you work with her by living a healthier lifestyle.

When possible leave the smog-filled, air-polluted cities for the country. In the quiet beauty of hill and meadow, you will rekindle your youth. To grow young again, believe you can, and strive and follow through for success. If you are a prisoner of a city, make it a point to go to parks, the country or the seashore where you can find true rest, tranquility, serenity and enjoy beautiful, recharging rest for your mind and body.

FOR HEALTHY, PEACEFUL LIVING

● **1.** Demand of yourself a higher standard of health and happiness. You cannot receive higher health unless your body gets its rest periods to develop new vitality and energy.

● **2.** Regard your body as a wonderful, miracle machine under your care and control. Recognize that every machine must have rest periods. Without sufficient rest health problems build up with nerve force depletion. The great majority of Americans are nervous, stressed out and unhealthy. Read the Bragg Nerve Force Book for building powerful nerves.

● **3.** As you grow older draw closer and more intimately to Mother Nature. Cease to look for thrills and over stimulation; instead, seek a life of serenity and peacefulness. Living in simplicity and purity you will have the healthy life Nature intended for you to enjoy for a long, active life.

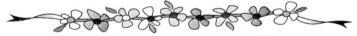

The natural healing force within us is the greatest force in getting well. – Hippocrates, Father of Medicine

---

Smile at each other, smile at your wife, smile at your husband, smile at your children, smile at each other – it doesn't matter who it is – and that will help you grow up in greater love for each other. – Mother Teresa

Let health, air, sun and peaceful rest work for you. With a serene, clear eye, and confidence, put yourself in Mother Nature's hands. Let her run your machine, heal your hurts, comfort you in sickness and adversity. Then, when you have lived a long life of usefulness and happiness, let her call you back home. Make her your partner, and when you are resting, relaxing, and building new energy, Mother Nature will always be there with her kind hand on your shoulder. So be a child of Nature, don't look for sophisticated thrills. Find your fun and diversion in relaxation and other pursuits that are simple, down to earth and one with Nature. Your rewards will be many: renewed health, a calmness of spirit and a new awareness of the perfect natural beauties that Mother Nature and our Creator have bestowed upon us so generously.

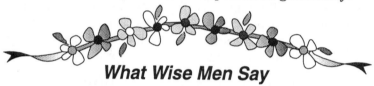

What Wise Men Say

Wisdom does not show itself so much in precept as in life - a firmness of mind and mastery of appetite. – Seneca

Health consists with Temperance alone. – Pope

Our prayers should be for a sound mind in a healthy body. – Juvenal

Govern well thy appetite, lest Sin surprise thee and her attendant Death. – Milton

I saw few die of hunger – of eating, a hundred-thousand. – Ben Franklin

Let nature be your teacher. – Wordsworth

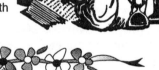

Diet caused diseases account for 68 percent of all the deaths in the United States. This means choosing the wrong foods is killing more Americans than infectious diseases, smoking, alcohol. drugs, accidents, traditional medical procedures, stress and the ageing process – combined.
– C. Everett Koop, Surgeon General's Report, 1988

Living is a continual lesson in problem solving, but the trick is to know where to start. No excuses – start the Bragg Healthy Lifestyle TODAY!

Chapter 15

DOCTOR GOOD POSTURE

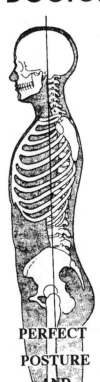

PERFECT POSTURE AND ALIGNMENT

Why should emphasis be placed upon such a simple thing as the pull of gravity? In your youth your muscles held your skeleton in proper balance free from strain or discomfort. Now, however, your muscles are losing the battle with gravity. Maybe you are prematurely older, or heavier, or perhaps an enforced rest has weakened your muscles just enough to its present uncomfortable state of balance.

This sagging stretches the ligaments of your back and causes backache. Ligaments that are stretched too far are painful. They are meant to serve only as check reins for the joints and cannot be forcibly stretched without pain. When the ligaments in your back are made uncomfortable by excessive stretching, it is natural for your muscles to try to oppose this gravitational pull. However, if your muscles are too weak to do their proper job, they will rapidly become exhausted and develop the misery of fatigue, making your back even more uncomfortable.

Check your own symptoms! Do you notice a deep aching and soreness along your spine due to stretched ligaments? Are your back and shoulder muscles achy and tired? Do you have a postural backache caused by weak muscles? If so, it's time you start to strengthen your muscles by proper exercise.

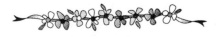

A strong body makes the mind strong.
– Thomas Jefferson

POSTURES

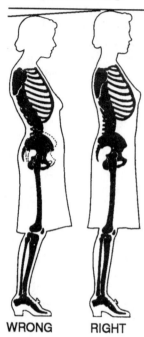

WRONG   **RIGHT**

Look at yourself in the mirror! Do your shoulders slump? Is your upper back round? Do you have you a potbelly? Are you swaybacked? Can you see the reasons why your back has the right to ache? The bending, slumping, ligament-stretching force of gravity has finally taken charge. Even though you might be a sufferer of backache due to poor muscles and bad posture, don't despair. With good exercise and posture habits you can most often regain back comfort!

It has been said that backache is the penalty people must pay for the privilege of standing and walking upright on two feet. Although some people believe our ancestors walked on all fours, it is an undisputable fact that we are definitely two-footed. Infants struggle instinctively to stand on their two feet and walk. They need not be taught! They attempt a bipedal mode even if left alone most of the time and never instructed. It is absolutely natural for human beings to stand and walk in this manner. This is especially interesting, in light of the fact that no other animals spend all of their standing and walking hours on two feet, not even the primates that are most like us, chimpanzees and the great apes.

These animals use their hands and arms to help move them about. The world's strongest gorilla would be unable to follow a fragile human about, walking erect on his legs, for more than a short time. This is because human beings are meant to walk erect and animals are not!

The spines of human beings have normal curves which enable the muscles to oppose gravity and hold their backs erect. As long as the muscles are strong enough to maintain the balance of these curves and prevent sagging, the back is comfortable. When the muscles are too weak to do their normal work, the back sags, ligaments are stretched, and often a backache is the inevitable result.

To maintain oneself in a healthy state involves many factors: healthy natural food, deep breathing, rest, exercise, sleep, control of emotions and mind, fasting, and good posture. If you nourish and care for your body, good posture is natural.

Conversely, when your body lacks any of the essentials, poor posture is often the result. Once you have established poor habits, you will have to take definite and corrective measures, You will need to exercise properly and practice good postural habits, in order to restore your natural, healthy state.

HOW TO STAND, SIT AND WALK
FOR STRENGTH AND SUPER HEALTH

When you sit, your spine should be straight against the chair and both feet should be squarely on the floor. Your abdominal cavity should not be relaxed, but well drawn in. Keep your shoulders back, and hold your chest and head high, never forward. Your arms may be relaxed or you may lightly clasp your hands in your lap.

When you walk, imagine that your legs are attached to the middle of your chest. This will give you long, sweeping, graceful, springy steps. When you walk correctly with this swing and spring, you will naturally build energy. **Habit either makes or breaks us, and good posture habits help make graceful, strong bodies.** *As the twig is bent, so is the tree inclined.*

When you are sitting, never cross one leg over the other. Under the knees run two of the largest arteries, carrying nourishing blood to the muscles below the knee and to all the nerves that are found in the feet. When you cross your legs, you immediately cut down the blood flow almost to a trickle. When the muscles of the leg and knee are not nourished and do not have good circulation, our extremities stagnate, which can lead to varicose veins or broken capillaries. Look at the bare ankles of people 40 and over who have made it a habit of crossing their legs and see the broken veins and capillaries. When the muscles and feet do not get their full supply of blood, the feet become weak and poor circulation sets in. And cold feet usually torment the leg-crosser.

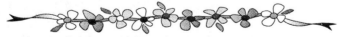

The quality of the blood depends largely upon its oxygenation in the lungs.
– Basic Physiology

A well-known heart specialist was asked, *When do most people have a heart attack?* He answered, *At a time they are sitting quietly with one leg crossed over the other.* When you sit, plant both feet squarely on the floor. Never cross your legs, because it puts an unnecessary burden on your heart.

People who are habitual leg-crossers have more acid crystals stored in the feet than those who never cross their legs. Crossing the legs is one of the worst postural habits of man. It throws the hips, the spine and the head off balance, and it is one of the most common causes of a chronic backache and varicose veins. Poor posture of any kind can bring an unbearable pain across your upper back, fatigue in your drooping shoulders, as well as soreness shooting from the base of your neck to the back of your throbbing head and downward to mingle with stiffness in your lower back. Poor posture can cause weakness in your hips and loins, a numb feeling at your tail bone, and, often, a shooting pain down your legs. Bad posture can develop aches and pains not only in the back, but all over the body.

CORRECT POSTURE IMPROVES HEALTH AND LOOKS

Establish this very simple, incredibly beneficial habit: stand tall, walk tall, sit tall. This doesn't require an exaggerated position. When this becomes a habit, the result is correct posture. All your sagging, prolapsed vital organs will slowly assume their normal positions and functions, if you daily follow the Bragg Healthy Lifestyle and practice good posture.

The doctor of the future
will give no medicine
but will interest his patients
in the care of the human frame,
in diet, and in the cause
and prevention of disease.
– Thomas A. Edison

Chapter 16

DOCTOR EXERCISE

Dr. Exercise makes this assertion, *To rest is to rust and rust means decay and destruction.* In other words, the good doctor tells us that **activity is life, stagnation is death.** The good doctor further tells us, that if we do not use our muscles, we lose them! In order to keep muscles firm, strong, vigorous, and youthful, they must be continually used. Activity is the Law of Life! Action is the Law of Well-Being. Every vital organ of the body has its specialized work, upon the performance of which its development and strength depend.

When we use the body, we build endurance, strength and vigor. Daily exercise promotes good blood circulation. When we become lazy and do not use our muscles the blood does not circulate as freely, the changes do not take place in it that are so vital to life and health. The muscles become flabby, sick, weak and unable to take vigorous activity.

People who do not exercise regularly have poor skin tone. When we exercise, we bring on healthy perspiration in the 96 million pores of our body. Skin is the largest eliminative organ in the entire body. If someone would shellac or gild your body and thus clog all your pores, you would die within a few minutes. With exercise, you bring on healthy perspiration.

Impurities and toxic poisons are expelled when you are exercising and perspiring freely, and you are allowing the skin to perform its natural function of eliminating poisons, If you do not exercise daily to the point of perspiration, all the work that the pores are not doing, throws a double burden on the other eliminative organs and then trouble occurs, physically. Vigorous exercise helps to normalize blood pressures and helps create a healthy pulse. Vigorous exercise is an anticoagulant, which means that it keeps the blood from forming the clots which often brings on a heart attack.

Every creature and humans seeking to eliminate the internal waste, does so by means of muscular action. Inside your intestinal tract there are three muscular layers which undergo a rhythmic, wavelike action called peristalsis.

If you allow the internal and external muscles, through inactivity, to become flabby and fat instead of muscular, the muscles lose their tone and power to contract, and the result is intestinal clogging. The abdominal muscles play an important role in the evacuation effort.

What happens when the internal and external muscles become flabby, weak, sick and infiltrated with fat? They often refuse to work, and intestinal waste piles up that should have been eliminated. This results in the buildup of large amounts of toxins. Inactivity is the cause of many diseases.

Fasting, and a healthy lifestyle are your friends in your pursuit of long-lasting youth, health and symmetry. When it comes to fighting fat . . . diet and fasting come first, but when it comes to keeping fit, it is exercise that matters most. However, they all help each other, for by taking exercise you may be more generous with your diet. The human machine should work well at the highest pitch of efficiency. All machines improve with intelligent use, and nothing betrays its weak spots like inactivity, rust, lack of maintenance and inadequate fuel. For example, your car's routine maintenance includes gas, oil changes, tune-ups, etc.

BRISK WALKING FOR HEALTHIER, LONGER LIFE

I recommend all of the many forms of exercise and participate in many. But without hesitation, I will tell you that walking is the best all-around exercise there is. Of all forms of exercise, brisk walking is the one that brings most of the body into action. As you walk, grasp yourself in the small of the back, and feel how your entire frame responds to every stride. Feel how almost all of your chief muscles are functioning rhythmically. In no other exercise do we get the same harmony of coordinating muscles and the same perfect circulation of blood.

Healthy Mind Habit: *Wake up and say – Today I am going to be happier, healthier and wiser in my daily living as I am the captain of my life and am going to steer it for 100% healthy living! Fact - Happy people look younger, live longer and have fewer health problems!* — Patricia Bragg

WALKING, THE KING OF EXERCISE IS IDEAL FOR YOU!

Walking should never be done consciously. No heel and toe business. No getting there in a certain time. Let it be, as it is, the most functional of exercises. Carry yourself well. Walk naturally with your head high and chest up. You will feel physically elated, and you will carry yourself proudly, straight and erect – and walk with an easy arm-swing.

Vow to become a wonderful walker, and make the day's walk a fixed item in your health program all the year round, and in any kind of weather. Go at your own stride with your spirit free. If the outer world of nature fails to interest you, turn to the inner world of the mind. As you walk, your body ceases to matter and you become part of nature surrounding you, and as near poet and philosopher as you will ever be.

Each to his taste, but to my mind this is better than golf. Life has so much to teach us that it is a pity to waste big chunks of time trying to get a ball into a hole in a stroke less than the other person. Most courses use electric golf carts which, unfortunately, eliminate walking time.

Gardening, too, is a marvelous form of exercise. It gives you exercise in the open air to help keep you in good physical condition. But you can get fat while gardening, because there is too little movement, and you are bent over instead of being erect. For this reason, I prefer walking. But perhaps some of both is best for you. Achieve your goals by applying your energy productively in your garden, then take the kink out of your back with a healthy brisk walk and some stretching.

Personally, I combine calisthenics with brisk walking, biking, swimming and tennis. I also enjoy my garden exercise and have 150 roses and an organic vegetable garden to enjoy.

IMPORTANCE OF ABDOMINAL EXERCISES

The most important exercises stimulate all of the muscles of the human trunk from the hips to the armpits. These are the binding muscles which hold all of the vital organs in place, for, in developing your torsal muscles, you are also developing the vital muscles. As your back, waist, chest and abdomen increase in soundness and elasticity, so will your lungs, liver, heart, stomach and kidneys gain in efficiency.

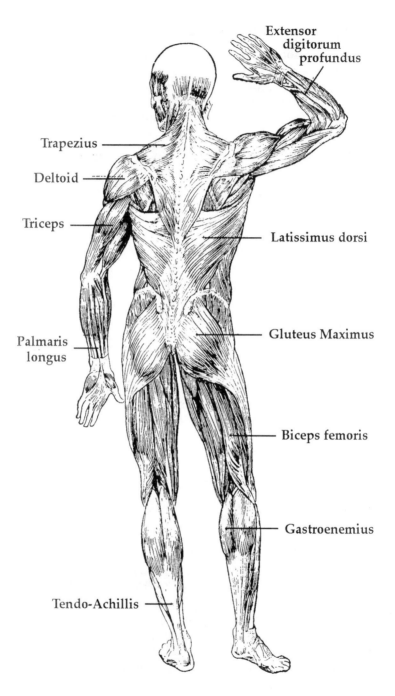

Extensor
digitorum
profundus

Trapezius

Deltoid

Triceps

Latissimus dorsi

Palmaris
longus

Gluteus Maximus

Biceps femoris

Gastroenemius

Tendo-Achillis

The muscles of the human body. Back view.

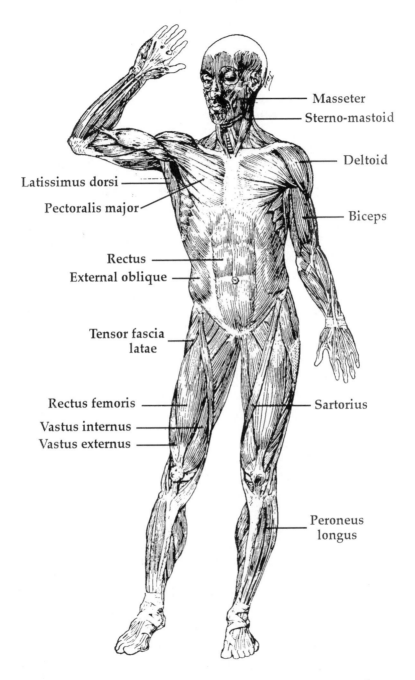

Masseter

Sterno-mastoid

Deltoid

Latissimus dorsi

Pectoralis major

Biceps

Rectus

External oblique

Tensor fascia
latae

Rectus femoris

Sartorius

Vastus internus

Vastus externus

Peroneus
longus

The muscles of the human body. Front view.

When you exercise regularly, the arch of your ribs widens. This gives free play to your lungs. Your elastic diaphragm allows the heart to pump and function more powerfully. Your rubberlike waist, in its limber action, stimulates your kidneys and massages your liver. Your abdominal muscles strengthen and support your stomach with controlled undulations. All of this trunk exercise is like a massage of the vital organs and it has an influence over the whole organism that must not be underestimated – it's vital!

SHALL WE EXERCISE DURING FASTING?

This is a question which only the faster can answer. If during a fast there is no inclination for physical activity, then you should not exercise. The fast is giving you a physiological rest and, unless there is a tremendous, overwhelming urge for physical activity, you should rest as much as possible.

During a fast your body is using all of its Vital Power for internal purification, but if you should feel, during a seven to ten day fast, that you need some stretching or walking, respond to the urge. It is between fasts and in your daily program of living that you should spend a portion of every day of your life, preferably in out-of-door exercises. Soon you will enjoy a vigorous circulation instead of a sluggish one. Sluggish circulation can cause many physical problems, discomfort, pain, and misery in the body.

The more you fast, the more poisons you will cleanse from your body. As your body increases in internal cleanliness, your muscles have more energy, tone and vitality. You will find that the old sluggish lazy feeling will leave you, and you will desire more action and more physical activity.

When people do not exercise, their ankles and legs often swell because there's not enough blood circulating to remove the waste from the cells and carry it back to the organs of elimination. There should be no excuse for not exercising. Regardless of your physical condition, it is vitally important that some exercise become a part of your healthy lifestyle.

Exercise helps avert sickness and premature ageing. It builds a health fund of endurance and resistance. It helps to build a healthy bloodstream with properly balanced white and red corpuscles that keep us healthy by fending off the many viruses and bacteria we are exposed to daily.

Exercise helps maintain a serene and tranquil mind and increases confidence . A one to three mile walk in the fresh air will help neutralize any unhealthful emotional upset you may experience. The knowledge that you have improved your mental and physical abilities through exercise will give you supreme confidence. Exercise helps cultivate the will and gives you control of your Physical, Mental, and Spiritual Self which helps you promote personal efficiency and happiness.

Exercise is the greatest health tonic we can provide ourselves! To attain this feeling of radiant, glorious health follow the Bragg Healthy Lifestyle. You will feel better and look better! A body that engages in regular, vigorous physical activity produces the miraculous feeling of agelessness.

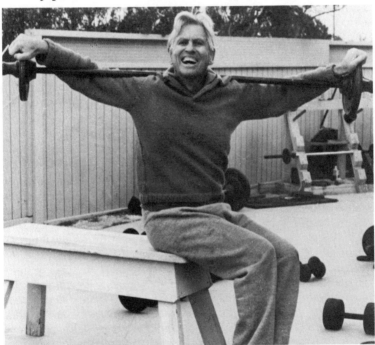

PAUL C. BRAGG WEIGHTLIFTED THREE TIMES A WEEK

Here he is at his outside gym in Palm Springs, California. Bragg was an early weightlifting pioneer. Weightlifting quickly reverses the loss of muscle tone and strength many people experience as they age and assume sedentary lives. A 93 year old participant in a weightlifting experiment with the elderly at Tufts University said, "I feel as though I were 50 again. Every day I feel better, younger and more optimistic."

HEALTHY HEART HABITS FOR A LONG, VITAL LIFE

Live foods make live people, and you are what you eat, drink and do, so eat a low-fat, low-sugar, high-fiber diet of whole grains and pastas, beans, brown rice, fresh salad greens, sprouts, vegetables, fruits, raw seeds, nuts, juices and six to eight glasses of distilled water daily.

Earn your food with daily exercise, for regular exercise improves your health, heart, flexibility and endurance, and helps open the cardiovascular system. Only 45 minutes a day can do miracles for your mind and body. You become revitalized with new zest for living.

We are made of tubes. To help keep them clean and open, make a mixture using 1/2 raw oat bran and 1/2 psyllium husk powder and add 1 to 3 tsp daily to juices, pep drinks, herb teas, soups, hot cereals, foods, etc. Daily I also take one Cayenne capsule (40,000 HU) with a meal.

Another way to daily guard against clogged tubes is to add 2 Tbsp soy lecithin granules [a fat emulsifier] to beverages, veggies, soups, etc.

Take 50 to 100 mgs regular-released Niacin (B-3) with one meal daily to help cleanse and open the cardiovascular system. Skin flushing may occur, nothing to worry about as it shows it's working! After cholesterol level reaches 180 or lower, take one to two Niacin weekly.

Your heart needs a good balance of nutrients, so take a natural vitamin-mineral food supplement with extra Vitamin E (mixed Tocopherols), Vitamin C, Magnesium, Selenium, Zinc, Beta Carotene & the amino acid L-Carnitine – your heart's super helpers! It's also wise to take a multi-digestant enzyme with each meal to aid digestion.

Also use the amazing antioxidants Pycnogenol (grape seeds) or SOD (super oxide dismutase). They help flush out dangerous free radicals that can cause havoc with your cardiovascular pipes and general health. Latest research shows they promote longevity, slow ageing, fights toxins, age spots, arthritis and its stiffness, swelling and pain, and help prevent cataracts, jet lag, exhaustion and disease.

Count your blessings daily while you do your 30 minutes or more brisk walk and exercises with these affirmations – *health! strength! youth! vitality! peace! laughter! humility! understanding! forgiveness! joy!* and *love for eternity!* – and soon all these qualities will come flooding and bouncing into your life. With blessings of super health, peace and love to you, our dear friends and readers.   – Patricia Bragg

RECOMMENDED BLOOD CHEMISTRY VALUES

- Total Cholesterol: 180 mg/dl or less; 150 mg/dl or less is optimal
- Total Cholesterol, Childhood Years: 140 mg/dl or less
- HDL Cholesterol: Men, 46 mg/dl or more; Women, 56 mg/dl or more
- HDL Cholesterol Ratio: 3.2 or less   • Glucose: 80-100 mg/dl
- Triglycerides: 100 mg/dl or less   • LDL Cholesterol: 120 or less

Chapter 17

DOCTOR SUNSHINE

Doctor Sunshine's specialty is heliotheraphy, and his great prescription is solar energy. Each tiny blade of grass, every vine, tree, bush, flower, fruit and vegetable draws its life from solar energy. All living things on earth depend on solar energy for their very existence. This earth would be a barren, frigid place if it were not for the magic rays of the sun. The sun gives us light, and were it not for light, there would be No You or Me. The earth would be in everlasting darkness. Humans were never meant to have pale skins.

Man's skin is gently tanned by sun and air, and will take on a darker pigment according to his original type. It has been found that under constant sun even redheaded people will tan. Pigmentation is a sign that solar energy has been transformed into human energy. Man can only gain health, vitality and happiness in the gentle, healing rays of the sun. The people who are indoors too long have a sallow ghostly-looking skin. That is why so many women hide their sun-starved skins with face makeup.

People who are starved of the vital rays of the sun have a half-dead look. They are actually dying for the want of solar energy. Weak, ailing, anemic people are usually sun-starved, and, in our opinion, many people are sick simply because they are starving for sunshine.

The rays of the sun are powerful germicides. As the skin imbibes more of these rays, it stores up enormous amounts of this germ-killing energy. The sun provides one of the finest remedies for the nervous person, who is filled with anxiety, worry, frustration, stresses and strains. When these tense people lie in the sunshine, its powerful rays give them what the nerves and body are crying out for, and that is relaxation.

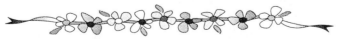

You are what you eat, drink, breathe, think and do!
What you eat and drink today will be walking and talking tomorrow!
– Patricia Bragg

99

Sunshine is a soothing tonic, a stimulant and above all, the Great Healer! As you bask in the warm, gentle sunshine (not the hot sun), millions of nerve endings absorb the solar energy and transform it to the nervous system of the body.

Make this experiment determine the value of sunshine in the matter of life and death. Find a beautiful lawn, where the grass is like a green carpet. Cover up a small space of that beautiful lawn with a small piece of wood or a box. Day by day you will notice that the beautiful grass that was full of plant blood, precious Chlorophyll, will fade and turn a sickly yellow. Tragically it withers and dies – death by sun starvation! The same thing happens in your body without the sun's life-giving rays and without an abundance of sun-ripened foods such as organic fruits and vegetables and their fresh juices.

We must have the direct rays of the sun on our bodies and we must eat at least 50 to 65 percent of food that has been ripened by the sun's rays. When we eat fresh, organically grown fruits and vegetables, we absorb blood of the plant, the rich, nourishing Chlorophyll. The life-giving chlorophyll is the solar energy that the plant has absorbed from the sun, the richest and most nourishing food you can put into your body.

CHLOROPHYLL IS MIRACLE LIQUID SUNSHINE

Green plants and vegetables alone possess the secret of how to capture this powerful solar energy and pass it on to man and every other living creature. When you put sunshine on the outside of your body, and eat ample raw, organic fruits and vegetables daily, you are going to glow with more super radiant health. But these powerful, natural remedies must be taken in very small doses at the beginning, because your sun-starved body cannot absorb too great an amount at first.

When you take your first sunbath, start with short time periods until you can condition your body to take more. The best time for a beginner to start taking sunbaths is in the early morning sunshine or the late afternoon sunshine. Five to ten minutes on the nude body is sufficient at first. The best rays of the sun are in the early morning or after 3 in the afternoon . . . these have the cooling rays. Between 11 to 3 we usually avoid the stronger rays of the sun. I'm known for the Hawaiian straw hats I wear, and I'm thankful for the shade they give my face when I'm in the hot sun.

100

The same caution should be taken in eating sun-ripened foods . . . the raw fruits and vegetables. The average person who has been eating mainly cooked foods will find that . . . if suddenly great amounts of raw fruit and vegetables are put into the body they can cause a reaction. It is wiser to gradually add more and more sun ripened foods to the diet. Overdoses of solar energy, both outside the body and in the body, are not good. In exposure to the sun, it is very important to use good judgment and proceed with caution.

When my father was diagnosed with tuberculosis at 16, the greatest doctors in the United States declared his case *Hopeless and Incurable!* But, by the Grace of God, he was led to Dr. August Rollier of Leysen, Switzerland, the greatest living authority on Heliotheraphy (Sun Cure). High in the Alps. His sick, wasting body was exposed to the healing rays of the sun and fed an abundance of natural, sun ripened foods.

A miracle happened. In two years he was transformed from a hopeless invalid on his deathbed to a vitally strong young man. At 95 years young he was still a powerful and healthy man. Through all those years, he continually exposed his body to the gentle, healing rays of the sun.

Dr. Healing Sunshine saved his life. That is why my father and I have always been worshipers of God's own precious sunshine. That is why we made our main home in California, the great sunshine state (except Los Angeles where the sickening smog has replaced the sunshine). We have a cabin high in the Santa Monica mountains so that we can get the benefit of the mountain sunshine. We have a modest home in the California Desert, where the sun shines 354 days a year.

We love the beach. We spent happy hours, winter and summer, on the great beaches of the world, Hawaii, Florida, at Cannes, France, Rhodes, Crete, Capri, Australia, New Zealand and Tahiti. I spend part of every year at my Hawaiian beach home, at the base of Diamond Head. Seek fresh, clean air and sunshine and Health will come by leaps and bounds and be yours to treasure!

Use your feet as nature intended. Give them every possible freedom. Go barefoot every chance you get.

Little things are like weeds – the longer we neglect them, the larger they grow.

Fasting has been rediscovered through juice fasting – as a simple, easy means of cleansing and restoring health and vitality.

To fast (abstain from food) comes from the Old English word *fasten* or *to hold firm*. It's a means to commit oneself to the task of finding inner strength through body, mind and soul cleansing. Throughout history the world's greatest philosophers and sages, including Socrates, Plato, Buddha and Gandhi, have enjoyed fasting and preached its benefits.

Juice bars are springing up everywhere and juice fasting has become "in" with the theatrical crowd in Hollywood and New York. The number of Stars who believe in the power and effectiveness of juice and water fasting is growing. A partial list includes: Steven Spielberg, Barbra Streisand, Kim Basinger, Alec Baldwin, Daryl Hannah, Christie Brinkley and Donna Karan. They say fasting helps balance their lives physically, mentally and emotionally.

Although a pure water fast is best, an introductory liquid juice fast can offer people an ideal opportunity to give their intestinal systems a restful, cleansing relief from the commercial high-fat, high-sugar, high-salt and high-protein fast foods too many Americans exist on daily.

Organic, raw, live fruits and vegetable juices can be purchased fresh from many Health Stores. You can also prepare these healthy juices yourself using a good home juicer. When juice fasting, it's best to dilute the juice with 1/3 distilled water. The list below gives you many combination ideas. With vegetable and tomato combinations try adding a dash of Bragg Liquid Aminos, herbs or, on non-fast days, even some green powder (barley, chlorella, spirulina, etc.) to create a delicious, nutritious powerful health drink. When using herbs in these drinks, use 1 to 2 fresh leaves or a pinch of dried herbs. A pinch of Dulse (seaweed), rich in protein, iodine and iron, is delicious with vegetable juices.

Here are some Powerful Juice Combinations:

1. *Beet, celery, alfalfa sprouts*
2. *Cabbage, celery and apple*
3. *Cabbage, cucumber, celery, tomato, spinach and basil*
4. *Tomato, carrot and mint*
5. *Carrot, celery, watercress, garlic and wheatgrass*
6. *Grapefruit, orange and lemon*
7. *Beet, parsley, celery, carrot, mustard greens, cabbage, garlic*
8. *Beet, celery, dulse and carrot*
9. *Cucumber, carrot and parsley*
10. *Watercress, cucumber, garlic*
11. *Asparagus, carrot, and mint*
12. *Carrot, celery, parsley and cabbage, onion, sweet basil*
13. *Carrot and coconut milk*
14. *Carrot, broccoli, lemon, cayenne*
15. *Carrot, cauliflower, rosemary*
16. *Apple, carrot, radish, ginger*
17. *Apple, pineapple and mint*
18. *Apple, papaya and grapes*
19. *Papaya, cranberries and apple*
20. *Leafy greens, broccoli, apple*
21. *Grape, cherry and apple*
22. *Watermelon (include seeds)*

Juicing has come a long way since Paul C. Bragg imported the first hand operated vegetable-fruit juicer from Germany and introduced juice therapy to America. Before this, juice was pressed by hand using cheesecloth. Juices are now considered an ideal health beverage worldwide!

FASTING – CLEANSES, RENEWS & REJUVENATES

Our bodies have a natural self-healing system for maintaining a healthy body and our "river of life" – our blood. It is essential that we keep our entire bodily machinery in good working order.

Fasting is the best detoxifying method. It's also the most effective and safest way to increase elimination of waste buildups and enhance the body's miraculous self-healing and self-repairing process that keeps you healthy.

If you prepare for a fast by eating a cleansing diet for 1 to 2 days, this can greatly facilitate the cleansing process. Fresh variety salads, fresh vegetables and fruits and their juices, as well as green drinks (alfalfa, barley, chlorophyll, chlorella, spirulina, wheatgrass, etc.) stimulate waste elimination. Live, fresh foods and juices can literally pick up dead matter from your body and carry it away. Following this pre-cleansing you can start your liquid fast.

Daily, even on some days during our fasts, we take 3,000 mg. of mixed Vitamin C powder (C concentrate, Acerola, Rosehips and Bioflavonoids) in liquids. It is a potent antioxidant and free radical scavenger. It also promotes collagen production for new healthy tissues. Vitamin C is especially important if you are detoxifying from prescription drugs, street drugs or alcohol overload.

A moderate, well planned distilled water fast or diluted juice (35% distilled water) fast can cleanse your body of excess mucus, old fecal matter, trapped cellular, non-food wastes and help remove inorganic mineral deposits and sludge from your pipes and joints.

Fasting works by self-digestion. During a fast your body intuitively will decompose and burn only the substances and tissues that are damaged, diseased or unneeded, such as abscesses, tumors, excess fat deposits, excess water and congestive wastes.

Even a relatively short fast (1 to 3 days) will accelerate elimination from your liver, kidneys, lungs, bloodstream and skin. Sometimes you will experience dramatic changes (cleansing and healing crisis) as accumulated wastes are expelled. With your first fasts you may temporarily have headaches, fatigue, body odor, bad breath, coated tongue, mouth sores and even diarrhea as your body is cleaning house. Please be patient with your body.

After a fast your body will begin to healthfully rebalance, when you follow the Bragg Healthy Lifestyle. The weekly 24 hour fast removes toxins on a regular basis, so they don't accumulate. Your energy levels will begin to rise – physically, psychologically and mentally. Your creativity will begin to expand. You will feel like a "different person" – which you are – you are being cleansed, purified and reborn. It's an exciting and wonderful miracle!

Fasting is Cleansing, Purifying and Restful. – Meir Schneider

103

A fast of three days or longer should be conducted under ideal conditions. You should be able to rest any time you feel the toxins passing out of your body. During this time you might feel some discomfort. You should rest and relax in quiet until the poisons have passed out of your body. It's best to be quiet, at peace and alone when possible. This brief period of discomfort will leave as soon as the loosened toxins have passed out of your body through the kidneys, lungs, skin, etc.

During the longer fast you should not tell others what you are doing. Why not? During the fast you must keep only positive thoughts of the cleansing and the renewing miracles happening in your body. Too often others who are ignorant about fasting will project onto you their own uninformed, negative thoughts.

Our fasting is such a very personal and quiet time that many years ago Dad went into the Santa Monica Mountains in California and bought a tract of land in the wilderness of the Topanga Canyon near Malibu where he built a retreat cabin, identical to Thoreau's at Walden Pond. In that natural seclusion Dad and I enjoyed the quiet and peace for our fasting time. If it is possible for you to get away to some secluded place and do your fast in nature with fresh air and solitude, you will enjoy better results!

There are also some very fine health spas in our country where all the conditions are perfect for a restful fast. Inquire at health stores for any in your area. Many of our Bragg students who fast regularly tell us that they use their vacation as a period of fasting and purification of body, mind and soul. Often they will go to some beautiful spot and rent accommodations and take their fast in seclusion. I am not saying that it's necessary to go away to fast from your home. It is your castle and hopefully you will be more at peace there. The Bragg family are all fasters, and when anyone of us is fasting, we have great consideration for each other. We have an agreement not to ask each other how we feel during the fast. Fasting is so personal that no one can do anything for you during the fast, so the best thing is not to discuss it with others.

> WHEN YOU ARE ON A FAST FROM 3 TO 10 DAYS OR MORE,
> YOU ARE REALLY ON NATURE'S MIRACULOUS OPERATING TABLE.
> Nature is ridding you of the waste, mucus, toxins
> and other foreign substances in your body.

Fasting is an effective and safe method of detoxifying the body.
Fast regularly and help the body heal itself and stay well.
– James Balch, MD & Phyllis Balch, CNC, *Prescription for Nutritional Healing*

BENEFITS FROM THE JOYS OF FASTING

Fasting is easier than any diet. • Fasting is the quickest way to lose weight.
Fasting is adaptable to a busy life. • Fasting gives the body a physiological rest.
Fasting is used successfully in the treatment of many physical illnesses.
Fasting can yield weight losses of up to 10 pounds or more in the first week.
Fasting lowers & normalizes cholesterol and blood pressure levels.
Fasting is a calming experience, often relieving tension and insomnia.
Fasting improves dietary habits. • Fasting increases eating pleasure.
Fasting frequently induces feelings of euphoria, a natural *high*.
Fasting is a rejuvenator, slowing the ageing process.
Fasting is an energizer, not a debilitator. • Fasting aids the elimination process.
Fasting often results in a more vigorous sex life.
Fasting can eliminate or modify smoking, drug and drinking addictions.
Fasting is a regulator, educating the body to consume food only as needed.
Fasting saves time spent marketing, preparing and eating.
Fasting rids the body of toxins, giving it an "internal shower" & cleansing.
Fasting does not deprive the body of essential nutrients.
Fasting can be used to uncover the sources of food allergies.
Fasting is used effectively in schizophrenia treatment & other mental illnesses.
Fasting under proper supervision can be tolerated easily up to 4 weeks.
Fasting does not accumulate appetite; hunger "pangs" disappear in 1-2 days.
Fasting is routine for the animal kingdom.
Fasting has been a commonplace experience since man's existence.
Fasting is a rite in all religions; the Bible alone has 74 references to it.
Fasting under proper conditions is absolutely safe.
Fasting is not starving, it's nature's cure that God has given us. – Patricia Bragg
　　　　– Allan Cott, M.D. *Fasting As A Way Of Life*

Spiritual Bible Reasons Why We Should Fast For A Healthier, Happier, Longer Walk with our Creator

3 John 2	Deut. 11:7-15,21	Luke 9:11	Matthew 9:9-15
Gen. 6:3	Gal. 5:13-26	Mark 2:16-20	Neh. 9:1, 20-24
I Cor. 7:5	Isaiah 58	Matthew 4:1-4	Psalms 35:13
II Cor. 6	James 5:10-20	Matthew 6:6-18	Romans 16:16-20
Deut. 8:3	John 15	Matthew 7	Zechariah 8:19

Dear HEALTH FRIEND,

This is a gentle reminder of the great benefits from *The Miracle of Fasting* that you will enjoy once you get started on your weekly 24 hour Bragg Fasting Program for Super Health! It's a precious time of body-mind-soul cleansing and renewal.

On *fast* days I drink daily 7 to 9 glasses of pure distilled water, some herb teas and you may have some diluted fresh juices. Everyday, even some fast days, you may add 1 Tbsp. of this mixture (1/2 oat bran and 1/2 psyllium husk powder) to liquids twice a day. It's an extra cleanser and helps normalize weight, cholesterol, blood pressures and helps promote healthy elimination. Fasting is the oldest, most effective healing method known to man. Fasting offers great and miraculous blessings from Mother Nature and our Creator. Fasting begins the self cleansing of the inner-body workings so we can promote our own self-healing.

My father & I wrote the book *The Miracle of Fasting* to share with you the health miracles it can perform in your daily life and it's all so easy to do – it's an important part of the Bragg Healthy Lifestyle.　With Love,

Paul Bragg's work on fasting is one of the great contributions to healing wisdom and the Natural Health Movement in the world today. - Gabriel Cousens, M.D., Author *Conscious Eating* and *Spiritual Nutrition*

LOCATIONS IN THE BODY
WHERE PAIN AND MISERY HIT HARDEST

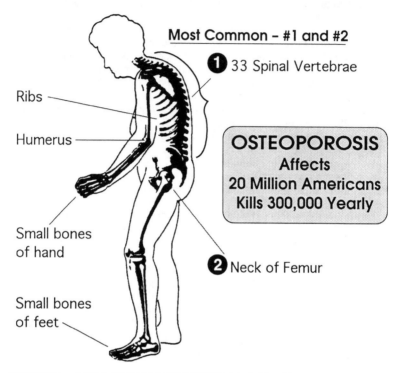

Most Common – #1 and #2

1 33 Spinal Vertebrae

Ribs

Humerus

Small bones
of hand

2 Neck of Femur

Small bones
of feet

OSTEOPOROSIS
Affects
20 Million Americans
Kills 300,000 Yearly

BORON – MIRACLE TRACE MINERAL FOR HEALTHY BONES

BORON – a trace mineral for healthy bones helps the body have more vital Calcium, Minerals and necessary Hormones! Good sources are broccoli, leafy vegetables, fresh and dried fruits, nuts, soybeans and nutritional yeast. The U.S. Dept. of Agriculture's Human Nutrition Lab in Grand Forks, North Dakota says Boron is usually in the soil and in foods, but many Americans eat a low Boron diet. They conducted a 17 week study which showed that a daily 3 mg. Boron supplement enabled participants to reduce the loss (demineralization) of Calcium, Phosphorous and Magnesium from their bodies. This loss is usually caused by most American's processed fast foods, consisting of high meat, high salt, high sugar and high fat diets.

After only 8 weeks on the Boron supplement, participants' Calcium loss was cut 40%. It also helped double certain important Hormones which are vital to maintain Calcium and healthy bones. Millions of women on estrogen-replacement therapy for Osteoporosis may use Boron as a healthier choice.

Scientific studies have confirmed that women benefit from a healthy lifestyle that includes ample exercise (to maintain healthier bones) combined with a low-fat, high-fiber, high-carbohydrate diet helps protect against heart disease, high blood pressure, cancer and more. Happy to see Science now agrees with my Dad who stated these simple health truths over 80 years ago.

106

FOOD AND PRODUCT SUMMARY

Today many of our foods are highly processed or refined, which robs them of essential nutrients, vitamins, minerals and enzymes; many contain harmful and dangerous chemicals. The research, findings and experience of top nutritionists, physicians and dentists have led them to discover that devitalized foods are a major cause of poor health, illness, cancer and premature death. The enormous increase in the last seventy years in degenerative diseases, such as heart disease, arthritis and dental decay substantiate this belief. Scientific research has shown that most of these afflictions can be prevented; and others, once established, may be arrested or even reversed through nutritional methods.

ENJOY SUPER HEALTH WITH NATURE'S FOOD

1. RAW FOODS: use food in its original state, organically grown whenever possible – especially fresh fruits, vegetables, whole grains, brown rice, beans, raw nuts and seeds.

2. VEGETABLE and ANIMAL PROTEIN:

    a. Legumes, soy and all other beans – *our favorites*.

    b. Nuts and seeds, raw and unsalted.

    c. Animal protein – variety meats, liver, kidney, brain, heart and poultry and seafood. Please eat sparingly but try the healthy vegetarian diet. You can bake, roast, wok or broil your animal proteins. Eat them no more than 3 times a week if you must.

    d. Dairy products, eggs (fer tile), unprocessed hard cheese and certified raw milk. (Personally we do not use milk and only occasionally unsalted butter and low or no-fat dairy yogurts.)

3. FRUITS and VEGETABLES: (organically grown is best – without the use of poisonous chemical sprays and fertilizers, – whenever possible); ask your market to stock organic produce. Steam, bake, saute or wok vegetables with distilled water, at low heat, for as short a time as possible.

4. 100% WHOLE GRAIN CEREALS, BREADS & FLOURS: they contain important B complex vitamins, vitamin E, minerals and the important unsaturated fatty acids.

5. COLD OR EXPELLER PRESSED VEGETABLE OILS: Olive, Canola, Sunflower and Sesame, are excellent sources of the healthy essential unsaturated fatty acids, but use sparingly.

PURE WATER - ESSENTIAL FOR HEALTH!

Distilled water is one of the world's best and purest waters! It is excellent for detoxification and fasting programs, because it helps cleanse and flush toxins and other harmful substances out of the cells, organs and fluids of the body!

Most water from chemically-treated public water systems, and even from many wells and springs, is likely to be loaded with harmful chemicals and toxic trace elements.

Too often the water in our homes, offices, schools, hospitals, etc., is overloaded with zinc or copper and cadmium from old water pipes. These trace elements are released in excessive quantities by the chemical interaction of water with the metals of the water pipes.

Pure water – either from the natural juices of vegetables, fruits, and other foods, or the pure water obtained by steam distillation or deionization – is essential for super health.

Your body is constantly working for you. It is 65% water and what you put in it will nourish you or kill you! Your body breaks down old bone and tissue cells and replaces them with new ones. As your body casts off old minerals and the products of broken-down cells, it must obtain new supplies of the essential elements in order to make healthy, new cells.

Scientists are beginning to understand that dental problems, different types of arthritis, and some forms of hardening of the arteries are due to imbalances in the levels of minerals in the body. Disorders can also be caused by an imbalance in the ratios of various minerals to each other.

Everybody requires a proper balance of all the nutritive elements in order to remain healthy. It is as bad for a person to have too much of one item, as it is to have too little of another. In order for calcium to be able to create new cells of bone and teeth, you must have adequate levels of phosphorus and magnesium. Yet, if there is too much of these minerals or too little calcium in the diet, old bone will be taken away but new bone will not be formed. Unbalanced and inappropriate diets can deplete the body of calcium, magnesium, potassium, and other major elements.

Diets high in meats, fish, eggs, grains, nuts, and seeds may provide excesses of phosphorus which will deplete calcium and magnesium from the bones and tissues of your body and cause these minerals to be lost in the urine.

High fat diets tend to increase the uptake of phosphorus from the intestines relative to calcium and other basic minerals. Such a diet can produce losses of calcium, magnesium, and other basic minerals in the same way a high phosphorus diet does.

Excesses of potassium in the body can be caused by diets too high in fruits and juices, and cause calcium and magnesium to be lost from the body through the urine.

Deficiencies of calcium and magnesium can produce many different problems ranging from dental decay and Osteoporosis to muscular cramping, hyperactivity, muscular twitching, sleep disorders and frequency of urination. Deficiencies of other minerals, or imbalances in the levels of those minerals, can produce many other health problems.

It is important to clean and detoxify the body through fasting and by drinking pure distilled water and healthy organically-grown vegetable and fruit juices. In order to continually provide the body with new supplies of minerals adults need to eat a diet containing wholesome organic vegetables, including kelp and other sea vegetables. Infants need only healthy mother's milk until six months of age.

Many adults and children in western civilization are malnourished and have low levels of essential minerals in their bodies due to losses caused by coffee, tea, carbonated beverages, and inadequate diets containing refined sugars and flours and table salt.

Additionally, the body's organ systems can be unbalanced by continuing stress, by toxins in our air, water and soil, by disease produced injuries and, in babies, by prenatal deficiencies in the mother's diet or lifestyle.

As a result, many people in our fast food society may need to take mineral supplements such as chelated multi-mineral supplements as well as a natural broad range multivitamin food supplement to ensure they get these vital nutrients.

The sense of obligation to continue is present in all of us. A duty to strive is the duty of us all. I felt a call to that duty. – Abraham Lincoln

FOOD FOR THOUGHT

Sir Isaac Newton, when writing his great work, "Principia," lived wholly upon a vegetable diet.

The word "vegetarian" is not derived from "vegetable," but from the Latin, homo vegetus, meaning among the Romans a strong, robust, thoroughly healthy man.

The health journals and the doctors all agree that the best and most wholesome part of the New England country doughnut is the hole. The larger the hole, they say, the better the doughnut.

The eating of much flesh fills us with a multitude of evil diseases and a multitudes of evil desires. – Porphyrises, 233 A.D.

The nervousness and peevishness of our times are chiefly attributable to tea and coffee. The digestive organs of confirmed coffee drinkers are in a state of chronic derangement which reacts on the brain, producing fretful and lachrymose moods. – Dr. Bock, 1910

The first wealth is health. – Emerson

An intellectual feast – Professor Louis Agassiz visited Germany to consult Oken, the transcendentalist in zoological classification. "After I had delivered to him my letter of introduction," he once said to a friend, "Oken asked me to dine with him, and you may suppose with what joy I accepted the invitation. The dinner consisted only of potatoes, boiled and roasted; but it was the best dinner I ever ate; for there was Oken. Never before were such potatoes grown on this planet; for the mind of the man seemed to enter into what we ate sociably together, and I devoured his intellect while munching his potatoes."

The world is moving so fast now-a-days that the man who says it can't be done is generally interrupted by someone doing it. – Elbert Hubbard

A physician recommended a lady to abandon the use of tea and coffee. "O, but I shall miss it so," said she. "Very likely," replied her medical advisor, "but you are missing health now, and will lose it altogether if you do not."

To work the head, temperance must be carried into the diet. – Beecher

110

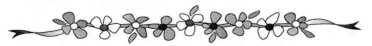

ALTERNATIVE HEALING HEALTH THERAPIES AND MASSAGE TECHNIQUES

Explore these wonderful natural methods of healing your body. Then choose the technique that's best for your needs:

F. Mathius Alexander Technique — Lessons intended to end improper use of neuromuscular system and bring body posture back into balance. Eliminates psycho-physical interferences, helps release long-held tension, and aids in reestablishing muscle tone.

Chiropractic — Daniel David Palmer founded chiropractic in 1885 in Davenport, Iowa. From 16 schools now in the U.S., graduates are joining Health Practitioners in all the civilized nations of the world to share their health-healing techniques. Chiropractic is the largest healing profession and benefits millions. Treatment involves soft tissue, spinal and body adjustment to free the nervous system of interferences with normal body function. Its concern is the functional integrity of the muscular skeletal system. In addition to manual methods, chiropractors use physical therapy modalities, exercise, health and nutritional guidance.

Feldenkrais Method — Founded by Dr. Moshe Feldenkrais in the late 1940's. Lessons lead to improved posture and help create ease and efficiency of movement. A great stress removal method.

Homeopathy — Developed by Dr. Samuel Hahnemann in the 1800's. Patients are treated with minute amounts of substances similar to those that cause a particular disease to trigger the body's own defenses. The homeopathic principle is *like cures like*. This safe and nontoxic remedy is #1 in Europe and Britain in alternative therapy because it is inexpensive, seldom has any side effects, and gets amazing, fast results.

Naturopathy — Brought to America by Dr. Benedict Lust, M.D., treatment utilizes diet, herbs, homeopathy, fasting, exercise, hydrotherapy, manipulation and sunlight. (Dr. Paul Bragg was a graduate of Dr. Lust's first Naturopathic School in the U.S.) Practitioners work with your body to naturally restore health. They reject surgery and drugs except as a last resort.

Osteopathy — The first School of Osteopathy was founded in 1892 by Dr. Andrew Taylor Still, M.D. There are now 15 such colleges in the U.S. Treatment involves soft tissue, spinal and body adjustments that free the nervous system from interferences which can cause illness. The complete system of healing by adjustment also includes good nutrition, physical therapies, proper breathing and good posture. Dr. Still's premise was that structure and function of the human body are interdependent and if the body structure is altered or abnormal, function is altered and illness results.

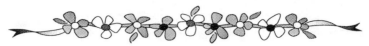

ALTERNATIVE HEALING HEALTH THERAPIES AND MASSAGE TECHNIQUES

Reflexology or Zone Therapy — Founded by Eunice Ingham, author of "The Story The Feet Can Tell," whose health career was inspired by a Bragg Health Crusade when she was 17. Relieves the body by removing crystalline deposits from meridians (nerve endings) of the feet by the therapist's using deep pressure massage. A form of Reflexology massage that has its early origins in China and is known to have been practiced by Kenyan natives and North American Indian tribes for centuries. Reflexology helps to activate the body's natural flow of energy by dislodging the collected deposits.

Reiki — A Japanese form of massage which means "Universal Life Energy." Reiki helps the body to detoxify, then rebalance and heal itself. Discovered in the ancient Sutra manuscripts by Dr. Mikso Usui in 1822.

Rolfing — A technique developed by Ida Rolf in the 1930s in the U.S., variously called structural processing, postural release or structural dynamics. It is based on the concept that distortions of nominal function of organs and skeletal muscles occur throughout life and are accentuated by the effects of gravity on the body. Rolfing helps the individual to achieve balance and improved body posture. Methods involve the use of stretching, deep tissue massage and relaxation techniques to loosen old injuries and break bad movement patterns which cause long-term body stress.

Self Massage — Paul C. Bragg often said, "You can be your own best massage therapist, even if you have only one good hand." Near-miraculous improvements have been achieved by victims of accidents or strokes in bringing life back to afflicted parts of their own bodies by self-massage and even vibrators. Treatments can be day or night, almost continual. Also, self-massage can help achieve relaxation at day's end. Families and friends can learn and exchange massages; it's a wonderful sharing experience. Babies also love and thrive with daily massages. Your family pets also love the soothing, healing touch of massage.

Aromatic Massage — It works two ways: The essence (smell) helps the patient relax as does the massage itself, while the massage is used to help absorption of essential natural oils used for centuries to treat numerous complaints. For example, Tiger Balm, Echinacea and Arnica help relieve muscle aches. Avoid creams and lotions with mineral oil because it clogs the skin's pores. Almond, avocado and olive oils are among the most popular. There are over 40 aromatics to use derived from herbs and other botanicals. (Pure rosemary oil, 6 drops to 6 ounces of olive oil is a favorite.)

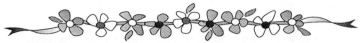

ALTERNATIVE HEALING HEALTH THERAPIES
AND MASSAGE TECHNIQUES

Shiatsu — It means *finger pressure* in Japanese and is applied with pressure from the fingers, hands, elbows and even knees along the same 12 meridian paths used in acupuncture (note: use only disposable needles!), which has been used for centuries in the Orient to relieve pain, common ills and muscle stress and to aid lymphatic circulation. This is a form of acupuncture – acupressure without needle punctures.

Sports Massage — Developed over the years into a sophisticated, important support system for athletes, professional and amateur. Sports massage serves these functions, AMTA says: improving circulation and mobility to injured tissue, enabling athletes to recover more rapidly from myofascial injury, reducing muscle soreness and chronic strain patterns. Soft tissues are freed of trigger points and adhesions, thus contributing to improvement of peak neuromuscular functioning and athletic performance. It is a preventive approach to injuries that can be suffered during training and it provides a psychological boost to athletes.

Tragering — Founded by Dr. Milton Trager M.D., who was inspired at age 18 by Paul C. Bragg to become a doctor. It is an experimental learning method which involves gentle shaking and rocking, suggesting a greater letting go, releasing tensions and lengthening of muscles for more body health. Tragering can do miraculous healing where needed in the muscles and the entire body.

Water Therapy — Showers are wonderful. First apply almond, avocado or olive oil to skin, then alternate hot and cold shower and massage needed areas while under shower. Garden hose massage is great in summer. Tub baths are wonderful as well: apply oil and massage. For muscle aches, add 1 cup of apple cider vinegar or Epsom salts. Dry skin brushing (brush lightly) is wonderful for circulation, toning and healing. For variety use a loofah sponge for massaging in the shower and tub.

Swedish Massage — Oldest and most-used massage technique. Deep body massage that soothes, promotes circulation and is also a great way to loosen muscles before and after exercise.

Author's Comment: My father and I have personally sampled many of these techniques. In 1994 health care bills soared to over $980 billion, and it is estimated that by the year 2000 they will reach $1.7 trillion. It becomes more important than ever that we take responsibility for our own health. This includes seeking holistic health practitioners who are dedicated to keeping Americans well by inspiring them to practice prevention. Many alternative healing therapies are becoming popular – massage, color, aroma, sound, music, biofeedback and yoga, to name a few. My advice to readers: Explore them and be open to improving your earthly temple for a long, happy life. Seek and find the best for your body, mind and spirit. – Patricia Bragg

HEALTH IS YOUR BIRTHRIGHT – PROTECT AND TREASURE IT

This is a priceless book. Please read and reread this book, until you get every health nugget it contains. Remember, you and you alone control your life, your health and the way you look, act, think and feel! Health comes from the inside out. You can be patched up after being stricken with disease, sickness and physical pain, but real 100% throbbing, vital health comes from good *health habits.* This book shows you how to turn away from the damaging, unhealthy living habits that fast living promotes.

It is now up to you to apply the intelligence that the Creator gave you. We teach simple, healthy living. You now have a treasure of knowledge of how to create a healthier, more joyful life through living this simple, healthy lifestyle.

Your health depends on your total lifestyle... the way you conduct yourself, each hour, each day, each week, each month and each year. You are the sum total of your habits. It is true that your body can take a lot of punishment from your bad habits. Sure, you can smoke, drink, eat dead, devitalized foods and apparently look and feel fine. Yes, for a while . . . but sooner or later you will have to balance your debts with Mother Nature! And when something breaks and you have heart trouble or one of the hundreds of other life and health destroyers – it may be too late. It may mean years of living death – or it may mean quick death.

We have no supernatural power to prevent or cure disease – that power is in your body. But modern science has discovered the way to live in health and happiness. We simply come to you as health teachers, to tell you in a simple, brief way what this healthy lifestyle can do for you. The rest is up to you. You have the knowledge; it is now up to you to apply the intelligence that the Creator gave you. This is simply common sense – and when something ceases to have common sense, it ceases to be scientific. You have a treasure here, and it's up to you to put it to use. This timeless knowledge of living a healthy lifestyle and being a super power breather will be a blessing to you.

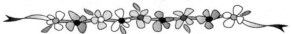

Living is a continual lesson in problem solving, but the trick is to know where to start. No excuses – start your health program today.

114

To attain this High State of Physical, Mental, Emotional and Spiritual Health practice Super Power Breathing and live the Bragg Healthy Lifestyle.

Be so strong physically and mentally that nothing can ever bring you back to an unhealthy way of living.

God bless you and give you the strength, the courage and the patience to reenter the Garden of Eden of Healthy Living.

With Blessings of Health, Peace, Joy and Love,

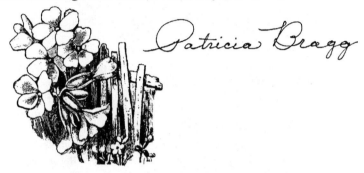

Patricia Bragg

*The Lord God formed man of the dust of the ground, and breathed into his nostrils **the breath of life**; and man became a living soul.*
– Genesis 2:7

Ten little two-letter words of action
If it is to be, it is up to me!

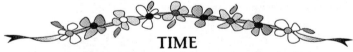

TIME

I have just a little minute, Only sixty seconds in it,
Just a tiny little minute, Give account if I abuse it;
Forced upon me; Can't refuse it. Didn't seek it,
Didn't choose it. But it's up to me to use it.
I must suffer if I lose it; But eternity is in it.

Many people go throughout life committing partial suicide – destroying their health, youth, beauty, talents, energies and creative qualities. Indeed, to learn how to be good to oneself is often more difficult than to learn how to be good to others. – Paul C. Bragg

The natural healing force within us is the greatest force in getting well.
– Hippocrates, Father of Medicine

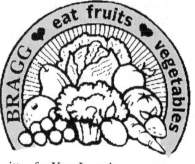
This book was written for You. It can be your passport to the Good Life. We Professional Nutritionists join hands in one common objective – a high standard of health for all and many added years to your life. Scientific Nutrition points the way – Nature's Way – the only lasting way to build a body free of degenerative diseases and premature aging. This book teaches you how to work with Nature, not against her. Doctors, nurses, and professional care givers who care for the sick try to repair depleted tissues, which too often mend poorly – if at all. Many of them praise the spreading of this new scientific message of natural foods and methods for long-lasting health and youthfulness at any age. To speed the spreading of this tremendous message, this book was written.

Statements in this book are recitals of scientific findings, known facts of physiology, biological therapeutics and reference to ancient writings as they are found. Paul C. Bragg practiced the natural methods of living for over 80 years with highly beneficial results, knowing that they were safe and of great value. His daughter Patricia Bragg worked with him to carry on the Health Crusades. They make no specific claims regarding the effectiveness of these methods for any individual, and assume no obligation for any opinions expressed in this book.

No cure for disease is offered in this book. No foods or diets are offered for the treatment or cure of any specific ailment. Nor is it intended as, or to be used as, literature aimed at promoting any food product. Paul C. Bragg and Patricia Bragg express their opinions solely as Public Health Educators, Professional Nutritionists and Teachers.

Experts may disagree with some of the statements made in this book, particularly those pertaining to nutritional recommendations. However, any such statements are considered to be factual, based upon the long-time experience of Paul C. Bragg and Patricia Bragg. If you suspect you have a medical problem, please seek qualified alternative health professionals to help you make the healthiest and wisest informed choices.

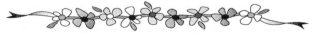

Prayer is the mortar that holds our house together. –Mother Teresa

SEND FOR IMPORTANT HEALTH BULLETINS

Let Health Science send you, your relatives and friends the latest News Bulletins on Health and Nutrition Discoveries. These are sent periodically. Please enclose one dollar for each USA name listed to cover postage and printing. Foreign listings please send international postal reply coupons. Print or type addresses, thank you.

HEALTH SCIENCE Box 7, Santa Barbara, California 93102 USA

●
_____
Name

_____ ( ) _____
Address   Phone

_____
City   State   Zip Code

- -

●
_____
Name

_____ ( ) _____
Address   Phone

_____
City   State   Zip Code

- -

●
_____
Name

_____ ( ) _____
Address   Phone

_____
City   State   Zip Code

- -

●
_____
Name

_____ ( ) _____
Address   Phone

_____
City   State   Zip Code

- -

●
_____
Name

_____ ( ) _____
Address   Phone

_____
City   State   Zip Code

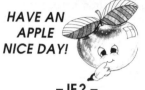
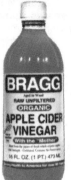

PAUL C. BRAGG N.D., Ph.D.

Life Extension Specialist • World Health Crusader
Lecturer and Advisor to Olympic Athletes, Royalty and Stars
Originator of Health Food Stores – Now Worldwide

For almost a Century, Living Proof that his
"Health and Fitness Way of Life" Works Wonders!

Paul C. Bragg is the Father of the Health Movement in America. This dynamic Crusader for worldwide health and fitness is responsible for more *firsts* in the history of Health than any other individual.

Here are Bragg's amazing pioneering achievements the world now enjoys:

- Bragg originated, named and opened the first *Health Food Store* in America.
- Bragg Crusades pioneered the first Health Lectures across America, inspiring followers to open health stores in cities across the land and now worldwide.
- Bragg introduced pineapple juice and tomato juice to the American public.
- He was the first to introduce and distribute honey nationwide.
- He introduced Juice Therapy in America by importing the first hand-juicers.
- Bragg pioneered Radio Health Programs from Hollywood three times daily.
- Paul and Patricia pioneered a Health TV show from Hollywood to spread *Health and Happiness*... the name of the show! It included exercises, health recipes, visual demonstrations, & guest appearances by famous, health-minded people.
- He created the first health foods and products and made them available nationwide: herb teas, health beverages, seven-grain cereals and crackers, health cosmetics, health candies, calcium, vitamins and mineral supplements, wheatgerm, digestive enzymes from papaya, herbs & kelp seasonings, amino acids from soybeans. He inspired others to follow and now thousands of health items are available worldwide.
- He opened the first health restaurants and the first health spas in America.

Crippled by TB as a teenager, Bragg developed his own eating, breathing and exercising program to rebuild his body into an ageless, tireless, pain-free citadel of glowing, radiant health. He excelled in running, swimming, biking, progressive weighttraining and mountain climbing. He made an early pledge to God, in return for his renewed health, to spend the rest of his life showing others the road to health. He honored his pledge! Bragg's health pioneering made a difference worldwide.

A living legend and beloved counselor to millions, Bragg was the inspiration and personal advisor on diet and fitness to top Olympic Stars from 4-time swimming Gold Medalist Murray Rose to 3-time track Gold Medalist Betty Cuthbert of Australia, his relative Don Bragg (pole-vaulting Gold Medalist), and countless other champions. Jack LaLanne, the original TV King of Fitness, says, *Bragg saved my life at age 15 when I attended the Bragg Crusade in Oakland, California.* From the earliest days, Bragg was advisor to the greatest Hollywood Stars and to giants of American Business. J. C. Penney, Del E. Webb and Conrad Hilton are just a few who he inspired to long, successful, healthy, active lives!

Dr. Bragg changed the lives of millions worldwide in all walks of life with the Bragg Health Crusades, Books, Tapes, Radio and TV appearances.

HEALTH SCIENCE, Box 7, SANTA BARBARA, CA 93102 USA

PATRICIA BRAGG N.D., Ph.D.
Angel of Health & Healing
Author, Lecturer, Nutritionist, Health Educator & Fitness Advisor to World Leaders, Hollywood Stars, Singers, Dancers & Athletes

Daughter of the world renowned health authority, Paul C. Bragg, Patricia Bragg has won international fame on her own in this field. She conducts Health and Fitness Seminars for Women's, Men's, Youth and Church Groups throughout the world... and promotes Bragg "How-To, Self-Health" Books in Lectures, on Radio and Television Talk Shows throughout the English-speaking world. Consultants to Presidents and Royalty, to the Stars of Stage, Screen and TV and to Champion Athletes, Patricia and her father are Co-Authors of the Bragg Health Library of Instructive, Inspiring Books that promotes the Bragg Healthy Lifestyle for a longer, vital, healthier life!

Patricia herself is the symbol of health, perpetual youth and super energy. She is a living and sparkling example of her and her father's healthy lifestyle precepts and this she loves sharing world-wide.

A fifth generation Californian on her mother's side, Patricia was reared by the Bragg Natural Health Method from infancy. In school, she not only excelled in athletics, but also won honors for her studies and her counseling. She is an accomplished musician and dancer... as well as tennis player and mountain climber... and the youngest woman ever to be granted a U.S. Patent. Patricia is a popular gifted Health Teacher and a dynamic, in-demand Talk Show Guest where she spreads the simple, easy-to-follow Bragg Healthy Lifestyle for everyone of all ages.

Man's body is his vehicle through life, his earthly temple... and the creator wants us filled with joy & health for a long fruitful life. The Bragg Crusades of Health and Fitness (3 John 2) has carried her around the world over 10 times – spreading physical, spiritual, emotional, mental health and joy. Health is our birthright and Patricia teaches how to prevent the destruction of our health from man-made wrong habits of living.

Patricia's been Health Consultant to American Presidents and British Royalty, to Betty Cuthbert, Australia's "Golden Girl," who holds 16 world records and four Olympic gold medals in women's track and to New Zealand's Olympic Track and Triathlete Star, Allison Roe. Among those who come to her for advice are some of Hollywood's top Stars from Clint Eastwood to the ever-youthful singing group, The Beach Boys and their families, Singing Stars of the Metropolitan Opera and top Ballet Stars. Patricia's message is of world-wide appeal to people of all ages, nationalities and walks-of-life. Those who follow the Bragg Health Books and attend the Bragg Crusades World-wide are living testimonials like ageless, super athlete, Jack LaLanne, who at age 15 went from sickness to Total Health!

Patricia Bragg inspires you to Renew, Rejuvenate & Revitalize your life with the "Bragg Healthy Lifestyle" Seminars and Lectures worldwide. These events are life changing, where millions have benefited with a longer, healthier life! She would love to share with your community, organization, church groups, etc. Also, she is a perfect radio and T.V. talk show guest to spread the message of health and fitness in your area.

Write or call (805) 968-1020 for requests and information:

HEALTH SCIENCE, BOX 7, SANTA BARBARA, CA 93102, USA